Cracking Your Calorie Code

Cracking Your Calorie Code

By PJ Glassey CSCS

Library of Congress Control Number: 2008904702
ISBN: Hardcover   978-1-4363-4508-8
                 Softcover   978-1-4363-4507-1

This book was printed in the United States of America.

To order additional copies of this book, contact:
Xlibris Corporation
1-888-795-4274
www.Xlibris.com
Orders@Xlibris.com
50612

CONTENTS

PROLOGUE

It was very difficult for society to accept the fact that the world was round at one point in our history. In the same way, nutrition, medical and fitness organizations are resisting the truth today. This book will explain to you the real facts, the current facts, and the truth about your metabolism and physiology.

You will learn how calories differ and how they affect you in a specific way and why they may affect someone else in another way. You will also learn how to understand your specific metabolism and how to crack its very complex code.

No one should have to hate what they eat to achieve the perfect body. No one should have to spend hours each week in the gym to achieve the shape they want. This is all sick and wrong! You have been fed only what you have had access to, and it's severely outdated. By contrast, this book is based on the latest studies.

There are many health, nutrition, and fitness books out there and most of them are written by "experts" who want to pontificate about their knowledge to the masses, and end up writing a diatribe consisting mostly of stuff we aren't interested in. Just because cellular muscle contractile processes interest me doesn't mean you will be equally fascinated or even want to know about it.

The first question you should ask is what qualifies me, the author, to answer these questions and write on these topics? My distinct advantage over other fitness trainers, doctors, nutritionists, and dieticians is that I have hundreds of current clients between my three personal training gyms and these people have asked me thousands of questions over the years since 1989 when I started my professional career.

I could provide most of the answers to these questions on the spot, and some I could not. The questions that do stump me are the most fun because it gives me a reason to research the answers which is my first love. Through this research, I found the answers to their questions and more. With every study I read, other related topics come to mind that spawn new research tangents. These sessions often snowball and birth new ideas and concepts for nutrition and exercise to add to my research and development list.

I also have a weekly radio talk show where callers ask me questions on fitness and nutrition. Listeners also email me during the week between shows with questions, comments, or topics they would like me to research for them.

Since I started my radio talk show, I haven't been stumped by a caller with a question on fitness and nutrition. There have been some tough questions, but from what I have learned over the years of studying the research, I have been able to provide the right answer to every question so far.

I don't claim to be a professional scientist but I do know how to read, understand and interpret research from my education and degree in Exercise Science. Since graduating from Seattle Pacific University in 1989, I have devoured the latest studies in nutrition and exercise. This journey has helped me develop several unique methods for strength training and cardio exercise without ever requiring more than 20 minutes per workout.

Everything in this book is backed by the latest studies and validated with repeat studies and correlated investigations. Since most of the ideas are based on multiple studies, the scientists are not listed with each reference. To list all the studies in this book, it would simply take up too much space. There is however, a full bibliography posted on the website *www.crackingyourcode.com* for anyone to browse.

I am a hopeless optimist so when I read some interesting new studies and come up with a new idea to try, I usually think it will be the best thing since sticky notes, and that it will completely revolutionize the industry. I enthusiastically dive into the trials with myself as the first test subject. More than half the time the method doesn't work as well as I had hoped, so I have to throw it away.

I figure if a new exercise method or nutritional concept doesn't work on me, it probably won't work for "most" other people either. It may indeed work on some and I'm sure I've passed up some good methods for a minority of the population in my single-mindedness, but I'm a pretty average guy, with pretty average genetics, and a pretty average metabolism, so if it works well on me, I figure it will probably work well on other people too. I also feel like I can enthusiastically promote that method or concept firsthand, without any hypocrisy or doubt.

The methods that do work on me are then tried on my friends and family. I have a buddy I have known since the third grade that is usually willing to give it a shot. My dad is always a willing test subject, and my trainers get as excited to try something new as I do. These test subjects are safe to use as guinea pigs because if it doesn't work, or might not be as safe as I had hoped, they don't get mad at me. More than half of those methods however, don't prove themselves better, so they are discarded. The ones that make it past these stages then go on to our X Gym members. More than half of those don't work either, so they are thrown out as well.

Most of the new methods we try do indeed produce better results than traditional methods, but the reason we throw them out is because they aren't better than the present methods we already have in place. To be adopted into our program and become a part of this book, a new method must prove itself markedly superior to one of the methods we are currently using. All of my ideas are pretty good, but you can see that most of them don't make it to adoption. In the end, less than two percent actually succeed in replacing one of our current methods. My new, great ideas that I get so excited about initially, fail 98% of the time!

Even though most of my ideas fail, I never feel discouraged or like I wasted my time, because I just figured out what doesn't work and can scratch that off the list. This list is very important because I can go back to it and avoid repeating the same mistakes. I can also refer back to it in case someone else comes up with the same idea later. Explaining why I think something doesn't work, backed up by my firsthand experience, is quite valuable to my clients and to you as readers. I have made all the mistakes for you already, so you can get right to the stuff that does work!

Most of the techniques used in the mainstream today were developed by someone with no research to back up their effectiveness. It just seemed like a good idea to them at the time so they went with it, and like many other ideas, it turned into the "thing to do."

In the 1930's, Joe Weider got a hold of Eugene Sandow's weight lifting techniques and with his publishing talents, made them mainstream. In 1951, Dr. Thomas L. DeLorme M.D. and Arthur L. Watkins M.D. published their book, promoting progressive weightlifting even further. Because of this momentum, we have continued with these outdated and invalid theories to this day, and steamrolled past what recent science has been trying to tell us along the way.

Most "fitness craze" ideas are created by individuals who come up with a good marketing idea but have no proof that it works. It's just a good persuasion item that will make you think it is effective, but it hasn't been properly tested or proven. They just market the concept or product to make a quick buck on the "suckers" and go away. The poor saps that buy into it simply waste their money and sink deeper into despair after experiencing yet another repeated failure.

Most infomercials use a few individual testimonials and case histories to "prove" their effectiveness. Case histories however, including my own, don't mean much when compared to research, because everyone is so different. My goal for doing everything first is to live through the experience personally so that I can help whoever is next as much as possible.

I feel like I don't have a right to tell someone where to walk unless I've already explored the path myself and found it to be a safe and worthy trail for others. It's only after an idea has proven effective with many others from a broad range of factors that it is worthy of adoption into my program or inclusion in this book.

Even health "professionals" are behind the times. Most nutritionists, dieticians and doctors are still outdated by at least 20 years because they are either too busy to do their own investigations into the latest findings, or they get caught up in the momentum of the colossal medical and dietary associations that take decades to change course.

Why do you keep trying the same thing over and over and failing at it every time? Ben Franklin once said, "The definition of insanity is doing the same thing over and over and expecting different results." It is now time to try something new that actually works! You can now stop wasting your time and start getting real results.

CHAPTER ONE

CRACKING THE RESEARCH CODE

In spite of the recent "fitness revolution" and being the most health-educated country in the world, Americans are fatter than ever. We even have the highest number of health clubs and personal trainers, but in spite of it all, we are still the fattest country on the planet. Most of the reason for this is because our knowledge is flawed and our mind-set is the opposite of what it should be.

You will of course gain knowledge by reading this book, but that alone won't help you much. Knowledge is just a tool. Most tools just sit in the garage and we forget we even have them. This book will show you truly new techniques that will help you use these tools so you can finally succeed with your fitness goals.

This book will show you why diets fail and fitness progress stagnates. You will discover the reason most New Year's fitness resolutions fizzle out by the end of February. You will finally, for the first time ever, learn new information that can make the difference you need for true and permanent change by changing the way your brain operates.

Science has discovered some pretty important things about us over the last 10-20 years, but few people are talking about them yet. Chances are, if you asked your trainer what new discoveries have happened lately, they will only be able to talk about what they have heard from others or read in the mainstream magazines. That information is still outdated by 50-100 years and skewed toward certain marketing to sell you products that just don't work.

The field of exercise science is very young. Scientific research on exercise didn't even start until the 70's and wasn't popular until the 80's. Even the studies from the 80's are often flawed because most scientists didn't know how to design them correctly, since they were all "pioneers" in the field.

When the 90's rolled around, they had enough experience behind them, and they started to get it right. The results from this research was so compelling, it motivated others to repeat the studies for confirmation and sparked new ideas for other studies. Most of the best information we now have is only 15 years old or less!

This new information shows us where we have gone wrong so far. It also shows us the direction to take to achieve the results we have been seeking for so long. This book is the first one published that explains these recent findings and dispels the myths in a way everyone can understand. It is your best shortcut to your goals so far. You will get results so fast, you will think you are cheating!

It is also important to note that everything I give as advice in this book has been personally tested by me on myself before anyone else. By experiencing weight gain, weight loss, and maintaining low fat levels while changing one variable at a time, I have found what works and what doesn't on a personal scale.

I am the first proof that these methods work. I am the leanest I have ever been in my life. Each year I feel younger, and I am the strongest I have ever been as well. My cardiovascular fitness increases every year, and my flexibility has also improved with age. I work out less each year, yet I feel in the best shape of my life and now look better than I have at any age.

Here is the real kicker: Even though I work out less each year as my age increases, I am eating the highest number of calories of my life. I was born in 1966, so it's pretty easy to figure out how old I am, but why am I getting younger physically as the chronological clock goes the other way? How is it possible that I am exercising less, eating more, and feeling younger every year? It is because I really have found out the new and better way to fitness! New research studies reveal further improvements every week, so I know I can look forward to even better fitness in the future.

Being an expert in the field of scientific research doesn't qualify me to write a book nearly as well as the fact that I'm wrong most of the time. I know that sounds contradictory, but the best scientists are the ones who get as much satisfaction out of being wrong as much as they do in being right.

Most scientists are hired by a company to conduct research that proves a certain point or theory. They are biased from the start, and no matter how hard they try to remain objective, they will usually be partial to their funding source. Their employer is providing them a paycheck to hopefully produce favorable findings for their product or idea. If the results of the study are negative, they are usually just buried and never published, or misinterpreted to show something that really isn't there.

Maurice Arthus, in his book *Philosophy of Scientific Investigation*, wrote quite eloquently, "In reality, those who repudiate a theory they had once proposed, or a theory they had accepted enthusiastically and with which they had identified themselves, are very rare. The great majority of them shut their ears so as not to hear the crying facts, and shut their eyes so as not to see the glaring facts, in order to remain faithful to their theories in spite of all and everything."

My job is not only to weed out the partial scientists and flawed and biased studies, but to test the ones I am doubtful of on myself and others to see firsthand if they really do work. Any time I come up with a new idea to test, I am very excited. I have high hopes that it will become the next breakthrough method, but most of them fall flat on their faces. In fact, more than 98% of the ideas I try end up failing miserably.

Luckily for me, I get just as much satisfaction out of my failures as I do seeing the few that do succeed come through on the other side. I don't mind failure because that allows me to cross a bad idea off the list. It is just as useful to avoid a bad method as it is to find a good one, because the bad method will waste as much or more of your time as the good one will save. You get to reap the benefits of my failures by skipping over what doesn't work and getting right to the methods that do work!

I have compiled these new discoveries into seven main "new facts." Most of these facts are considered blasphemy to the old school nutritionists, fitness "experts", and medical professionals, but that is only because they aren't as current with the recent research as they should be, or because they are biased. The recent wealth of new scientific information on fitness and nutrition proves almost everything we have been doing up until now has been wrong!

New fact number one: All calories are not the same. Nutritionists and dieticians will tell you that the number of calories you eat and the number of calories you burn will dictate whether you lose weight or not. I will explain why this is not true and that not only does the *type* of calorie matter, but the *timing* of certain calories matters as well. This all makes a huge difference in your weight gain or loss.

New fact number two: Food manufacturers are purposely including unnecessary ingredients in their products that cause you to become addicted. This addiction unfortunately, also leads to weight gain. In the movie "Supersize Me" it took filmmaker Morgan Spurlock a month to gain

30 pounds, but it took him a year to get the weight back off because of the toxins and preservatives stored in his liver and fat cells.

New fact number three: Weight loss doesn't have to be a matter of willpower. You will learn specific brain techniques that can eliminate the need for willpower to control cravings and addictions. You will also learn how to curb cravings and refocus habits into fat burning techniques instead of your present fat storing methods, which you might not even be aware of.

New fact number four: The metabolism you were born with is not permanent. It can be changed and even reset! Your new metabolism can even be handed down to your kids to give them an edge so they don't have to try as hard as you did! You will also learn how your metabolism can change from hour to hour, and how to control and manipulate it to your advantage. I will also teach you how to increase your metabolism through a simple change in attitude.

New fact number five: Traditional strength training was invented in 1891, so that should be obvious how outdated it is now. Why is it so hard for us to give up these archaic techniques? Why do most of us keep trying the same things over and over even though they haven't worked the way we need them to for over 100 years? You will learn why, as well as new strength training techniques that will cut your time from the typical strength training requirement of three times a week for an hour, down to 20 minutes, twice a week.

New fact number six: Conventional cardiovascular exercise is a waste of time. No longer will you be doomed to plod along for hours on the treadmill each week or frequent the overcrowded sweaty aerobics class. New research points to cardio methods requiring no more than 20 minutes per workout (or less) to blow away the results of hour long sessions of traditional cardio.

New fact number seven: Your biggest enemy and reason you have not achieved your goals is due to your own brain wiring. This is never addressed with traditional training or nutrition, so it should seem like a foreign concept to you, but hear me out. I listed this last, not because it is the least important, but because it is the most important. It is so important, in fact, that I have made it the first section in this book. So get ready to change your brain!

CHAPTER TWO

CRACKING YOUR MENTAL CODE

This section will be your biggest key to success. The rest of the book contains truly new ideas and concepts on calories, your metabolism, fitness, nutrition and more, which will produce double the fitness results you are used to in about ¼ the time. You will also see your plateaus disappear. Without this section however, it will just be adding new knowledge, and that alone won't help you much.

This section will be a recurring theme through the rest of this book and will be referenced often in context to the subject at hand. It is vital to read this first and re-read it if needed, so you can understand it thoroughly and apply it anywhere and anytime with any method or theory. The other sections can be read out of order as long as this one is understood first.

The main reasons that keep you from achieving your goals have very little to do with your body or metabolism and everything to do with your brain wiring. This wiring is worse in some and better in others, but can be fixed in anyone. It is the way nerve impulses travel along the branches you have formed that dictate how successful you will be in your health and fitness goals.

Have you ever started a diet with all the good intentions in the world, but then sabotaged it before you even knew what had happened? Your behavior can't be explained other than "old habits die hard." The real reason for the failure is that your subconscious mind hasn't yet received the message of your new good intentions.

Your subconscious mind is in control of your habits and actions. It also controls your physiology and metabolism more than your conscious mind. Your body will always follow what your subconscious believes. If it believes you are a fat person, you will be a fat person. If it believes you are a lean person, you will be that instead.

Your subconscious mind is very literal and therefore quite easy to train, so it important to phrase things correctly when you are programming it.

It does whatever it hears the most, so the messages you send it with your conscious mind will win by a simple majority.

You may find yourself thinking thoughts about being a fat person, but if you are thinking about being a lean person 51% of the time, your subconscious will buy into that and make it happen. Even if your conscious mind doesn't believe the majority messages you are sending, your subconscious mind will!

You can demonstrate this phenomenon to yourself with a very simple experiment. Next time you wake up cranky, have road rage, or are just having a bad day, say the words, "I'm happy." You won't feel happy, but if you say it over and over, pretty soon a happy thought will pop into your conscious mind. This is your subconscious hearing the message and then acting on it.

Your subconscious will always strive to prove itself right. It will even make sure it wins over your conscious mind. Since it only acts on nouns, it will make happen whatever you are emphasizing. If you say, "I don't want to be such a fat slob" It will act on keeping you a fat slob.

Your conscious mind may truly not want you to be a fat slob and although your conscious intentions are pure and sincere, your subconscious mind is getting the wrong message and is carrying out the wrong goal. If your wording is emphasizing the positive goal instead, your subconscious will work with you to make that happen. By telling yourself, "I will get leaner today" your subconscious will hear that and prove itself right by causing you to make different conscious and unconscious decisions all day to achieve that objective.

Getting these messages to your subconscious is about rewiring your brain. Over time, you will actually change the neural pathways in your brain, but it takes practice. You will not feel very good at this in the beginning, but with practice and diligence, you will build the skill and guarantee your own success.

Without an effective rewiring job, you will probably fail the same way you always have before, in spite of the highly effective methods and concepts in this book. The good news is that your nerve impulses can be easily rerouted to cause your success. After effectively rewiring your brain, you will find the right choices to be easy and even automatic in most cases.

Recent ground-breaking research has proven that there are easy and effective techniques to permanently change your wiring and train your subconscious. These techniques involve only five steps for the entire process. Some of the steps may not sound new to you and others will, but it is the combination of the steps in the correct order that make them the key to your success.

Each step has a specific action designed to be a tool you can use to master that step. Practice will produce the desired results so don't expect to be an expert right away. It is a process, and while some adapt quickly and others take more time, you can be confident that it will completely ensure your permanent success.

Most health and fitness books start with the feet and get you exercising first. They work their way up but stop at the neck and never address the cause of repeated failure. This book starts with your head and works its way down, so the results are permanent and the body you want remains with you for life.

There is one main reason people yo-yo with their diets. The rebound happens because when an individual does lose the weight physically, they are still the same person in their brain and have not changed their perception of themselves. This perception dictates old habits and even controls the metabolism to a significant extent. Even though they are now thin, their subconscious still sees them as fat, and because of that picture, they make conscious and unconscious decisions each day to fulfill that prophecy.

Your metabolism can actually be regulated by your perception. If you think you have a slow metabolism, you will create that physically. You will also use that as an excuse to eat the wrong foods and "give up' on fitness. I know it sounds crazy, but just changing the way you think about your own metabolism will make it go up without doing anything else!

Have you ever noticed how your friends who are wired and energetic are usually thin? The nervous or high strung ones are typically that way too aren't they? Now think of how sluggish and tired your obese friends are. The same goes for other animals besides humans. How many fat Chihuahuas do you see? How many thin hippos are there?

It can be a simple matter of cause and effect! If you think your metabolism is slow, you are going to act the part, slow down, and gain fat. If you convince yourself your metabolism is fast, you will follow that with action as well.

If you start to think of yourself as someone who has a high metabolism, you will cause the hormones and cellular processes to physically change. Emotional state is more significant than even scientists realize. Science will discover this in about 10 years and it will be mainstream in about 20 years (with the help of this book), but you are getting the information now!

Good examples of this phenomenon can be seen in everyday life. I can think of two right off the top of my head. The first example comes from one of the trainers who works for me. I expressed my concern to her yesterday that it looked like she was getting too thin. She answered back that she was indeed, and there was nothing she could do about it. She was eating like a champ (twice her normal amount), but because of the current emotional stress in her life, her body was burning food faster than she could take it in.

Another example happened just 40 minutes ago. As I am typing this, I am on an airplane. We were delayed on the tarmac due to an electrical issue. As soon as the captain explained there would be a further delay, the stress level went up among the passengers. This increased stress elevated their metabolisms and more than a dozen arms reached up to turn on the air vents over head. They were getting hotter because their metabolisms were increasing simply because of emotional response!

We are electrical beings. Our hearts and brains run on electricity. Our very atoms are electrical as well, with electrons spinning around at different speeds. Emotions can speed up metabolic processes and even the belief in a slow or fast metabolism can speed up or slow down the electron rate in our atoms.

I have a machine at my gyms that can measure my clients' metabolism from the oxygen and carbon dioxide they exhale. It is a very accurate measure and produces readings that can even tell me if they are a sugar burner or fat burner by nature. When testing them, I have to make them understand that to accurately assess their metabolic rate, they must relax as much as possible.

I leave the room for a while and come in to check the computer after about 20 minutes, hoping to see a good enough graph to stop the test. Even my entering the room causes a spike in metabolic rate. Other spikes might be from the client remembering something they have to do that day, hearing a noise outside the door, or thinking a stressful thought.

This confirms to me how dynamic our metabolisms really are and how much they are affected by our minds and situations. You really can change your metabolism with your brain, even if you were born with a slow metabolism, or have created that for yourself over time.

With the brain techniques you will learn in this chapter, you will be able to adjust your metabolism like a thermostat and even change it permanently. Other physical and nutritional metabolic changing techniques will follow later in the book, but starting here with the brain is the most important step, and the one that will change your metabolic rate the most.

I'm sure you have heard of the term "mind's eye." Pay careful attention to this concept because your mind's eye is the most powerful thing about you, and will dictate and control your continued success. You really have two mind's eyes. One is located in your conscious brain and the other in your subconscious brain.

Your conscious mind's eye is how you think you look. Your subconscious mind's eye is how you believe you look. Aligning the two will dictate how you turn out. If you change your mind's eyes while you are changing your body, you will be a different person in both ways when you achieve the body you want. This will make you stay lean and hold onto your new body instead of rebounding back to where you were.

Those who lose the fat and keep it off have changed their mind's eyes and think of themselves differently when they reach their goals. Those who don't change their mind's eyes will most likely rebound and continue the endless yo-yo. It really is that simple as a concept, but it is a learning experience and takes mastering the skill to get it right.

Your mind's eyes can even dictate your health and susceptibility to disease. A recent study determined that people who believe themselves to be treated unfairly are more likely to suffer a heart attack or chest pain. Study participants who believed they had experienced the worst injustice were 55 percent more likely to experience a coronary event than people who thought life was fair.

Those who reported low levels of unfair treatment had a 28 percent higher risk of heart problems than those who reported none, and those who reported moderate unfairness saw a 36 percent greater risk than those who reported none. [*Journal of Epidemiology and Community Health, Vol. 61, No. 6, June 2007: 513-518*]

Your body will follow your subconscious mind's eye every time. This section will get your mind ready to change, so pay the closest attention to the following five steps. As your conscious brain rewires your subconscious brain, you will notice other positive changes in your life as well. People around you will see your attitude change and your personality improve. Your relationships might even change for the better.

To some, this might be scary because their present mind's eye is very strong. You might see yourself in a certain way and have formed a deep rooted identity in that person. Even positive changes might be uncomfortable for you, but remember that practicing the following principles forms new skills over time and makes all that better as well!

You are in effect brainwashing yourself with these techniques. Most of us think of brainwashing as a negative thing and something to be avoided, but if it is for the better and to improve your health, it is a great thing!

You have already brainwashed yourself with negative nerve pathways over the course of your life until now, so it is time to reverse that process and get it right. The good news is that with regular faithful practice, you can create your new brain rather quickly and it doesn't take another lifetime to do it!

The other good news is that you don't have to believe this will work. It will be effective in spite of your own pessimism. It will, of course, work faster if you do believe it, but plenty of people have been brainwashed against their will, so you can make it happen simply with enough practice and repetition.

Your subconscious mind's eye might even change its perception before your conscious mind does. In this case, you will see fitness results before you expect them because it is working without you even knowing it. That's great! Keep up the good work, and pretty soon the conscious and subconscious will line up together for a permanently rewired brain.

Mind's Eye Step One: Visualize the body you want.

Cut out a picture of who you want to look like. You may already have this person in mind. Make sure your choice is a similar body type (height, race, proportions, bone structure, etc.) and that they are a healthy person (not too skinny, etc.) with no cosmetic surgical alterations.

Next, have a friend confirm those three points. Instruct your friend to withhold their opinion either way on how realistic this goal is. Simply ask them to answer the three criteria above. The more opinions you can get the better—especially from the friends you consider optimists.

Post this picture somewhere you will see it often. Cut off the head and picture yours there. When you do that, visualize your face the way you want it to look as well. If you imagine yourself thin, you will become thin. If you imagine yourself fat, you will stay fat. It really is that simple.

Every time you look at this picture, imagine how that feels now, in the present tense. Don't think about how nice it would be, or "what if", but picture how it feels right now. Instead of visualizing getting thin, visualize being thin. It should be fun to do this action and it should never be a chore.

This will be easier for some and harder for others, but each time you do it you will get better at it and will be honing your skill for imagination.

> *"Imagination is everything. It is the preview to life's coming attractions."*
> —Albert Einstein

The picture is just a reminder to do the exercise in the first person, so close your eyes while you are practicing. Picture looking down at yourself and seeing that body and enjoying how that feels. Looking at the picture during the exercise is not the same process because this is like looking in a mirror or through a window. That is practicing second person visualization and will not activate the same neural pathways.

First person visualization is teaching your subconscious that you already are that way, and when your subconscious mind's eye believes it, things really start to change. Lean people make decisions to stay that way, and fat people make fat decisions. If your subconscious believes you are lean, it will help you make different decisions and over time, willpower will no longer be necessary.

When you imagine how you want to be as if it has already happened, you are traveling specific nerve branches in your brain that are literally turning you into that person. Some of these branches have been traveled before, but most are being created for the first time. One a branch is created, it can be accessed again. The more it is accessed, the deeper it becomes, until accessing and traveling it are a natural occurrence even without conscious thought.

If you can't picture yourself a certain way, you will find it nearly impossible to become that way. The brain has to go there first for the body to follow. Most people try to change their body without first preparing their mind, and this is the main reason for repeated failures and backslidings.

Every Olympic gold medal winner pictured themselves on the podium and imagined how that would feel before they got there. Every billionaire believed in their subconscious mind they would be one before they made their first billion. In the same way, no one has become thin by surprise or woken up one day and unexpectedly exclaimed, "Wow! Look at me! I'm in the best shape of my life!"

If you imagine yourself looking the way you want to, you are much more likely to become that person. If you imagine yourself the way you are, you will likely stay that way. It's like playing a DVD in your brain, but with you as the star. Play the movie of the positives, and run the film as yourself looking through your own eyes.

Every time you catch yourself focusing on your fat, stop that DVD and put the lean DVD back on. Hone this skill with frequent practice. It only takes a minute or two to visualize, and if you are having a hard time, just know that it will get better and easier each time you practice. Celebrate your success and ignore the times you might fail. Failure is always who you were, not who you are. Success is who you are and who you will be if you think that way.

We have all made goals before and maybe even written them down, but posting them to remind ourselves every day and experiencing them in the present tense is vital to achieving them. More than 94% of New Year's resolutions fail because the goal is not visualized and rehearsed. People often picture the goal initially and even dream about its achievement when they make the resolution, but that is where it typically stops. They think about it as "wouldn't that be nice" instead of experiencing the goal as if it has already been achieved.

I had an overweight client who had four months until her wedding. Her goal was simple. She merely wanted her collarbones to show in the wedding dress she had picked out. She focused on this and imagined it daily. She rehearsed what it would look like and pretended to feel the experience of walking down the aisle with those bones showing. Sure enough, by the wedding day, that had happened.

Mind's Eye Step Two: Concentrate on the foods you should eat.

This same principle goes for nutrition. Focusing on what you should avoid eating will cause your subconscious to make you crave those foods. Focus instead on what you should be eating. If you do eat something off your plan, say, "That's not who I am," and switch your focus to who you are now and the foods you should eat next.

Adam and Eve focused on what they shouldn't do and look where it got them! They had so much good to focus on, but the one thing that was forbidden was the thing they obsessed over and allowed to take them down. We are all like that naturally, but this tendency can be changed and even reversed.

When a child is screaming, the parent usually says, "Stop screaming." This may or may not work, but even if it does, it will do little to prevent it in the future. The focus was still put on the screaming. If the parent instead says, "Use your inside voice" or "Please be quieter", the child will be more likely to comply and has been given a tool to learn better behavior next time.

Every time you tell yourself not to eat a certain thing, you are strengthening the very nerve pathway you are trying to erase. The more you think about not eating it, the more powerful that pathway becomes until it is even more powerful than before. This is how addictions form and deepen.

Before you start a diet, you eat a certain "bad" food a couple of times a day. You probably think about it a couple of times a day as well. The brain travels the same branch whether you eat it or think about it. As far as the brain is concerned, you either ate that food four times that day, or just thought about it four times that day. There's no difference because it's the same nerve pathway.

Now you start the diet and forbid yourself that food. Your willpower seems pretty strong at first and you don't have much trouble resisting. During the first couple of days you think about it eight times. Then each day you think about it a few more times, until a couple of weeks later you are thinking about the food you can't have 20 times each day. Now it's a willpower struggle because as far as the brain is concerned, you ate that food 20 times every day and the nerve pathway is deeper and stronger than ever before.

When the diet comes to an end or you give up, that addiction is much worse than before, even though you haven't touched the food at all! Most physical addictions last only a few days, but as you can see, mental addictions are much stronger. It's the mind and how we program it that dictates our success or failure.

If you redirect your focus by thinking about the foods you *should* eat, you gradually take power away from the other foods and after a while, your cravings will shift to the foods you are focusing on. I have seen this many times with many people, including myself.

I used to allow myself a cheat day every week. I used to focus all week on what I would eat that day and this caused many struggles. I would make it through the week on sheer willpower. I was ingraining my negative nerve pathways deeper six days a week even though I wasn't physically eating those foods on those days.

When I switched my focus to what I should be eating during the week instead, **the willpower issue was virtually eliminated**. I was now ingraining the positive nerve pathways six days a week and when I did get to the cheat day, it was like my past good days because the healthy foods were so ingrained and my desire for the cheat foods had lost their power. Even when I "binged" on my cheat day, it was still better than most other people's good eating days!

The mind can multitask well and switch between many different thoughts per second, but it cannot have two thoughts at the same time. Any thought we have is just a particular nerve pathway being traveled. Memories, emotions, visualization, etc. are all just nerve impulses traveling specific routes. The way that impulse branches off makes it a unique thought. Since the mind can only fire one impulse at a time, you effectively deactivate all other pathways every time you activate one you want to have.

All nerve pathways are either getting stronger and deeper, or weaker and shallower. They never stay the same. If you use a certain pathway, you are making it stronger and making it easier to access later. If you are not using a pathway, it is atrophying and getting weaker. This is how we forget things. The nerve pathway has been traveled so little, it atrophied to the point that access is difficult to impossible.

When you think of the food you should be eating, you are making that pathway stronger and atrophying the negative pathway simultaneously. You are curing your addictions and cravings to the foods you shouldn't be eating and creating cravings for the foods you should be eating at the same time!

Mind's Eye Step Three: Imagine your physical goals.

Write down how you want to feel physically and what you want to do. Resist the temptation to write down phrases like, "I want my knees to stop hurting" and replace it with "Strengthen and heal my knees." All goals must be positive phrasing and toward your end result.

This step is similar to step one, but instead of imagining how you want to look and how that feels, you are now imagining what you want to do and how that feels. Rehearse these experiences in your mind and enjoy them mentally. So what if you weigh 400 pounds want to learn ballet! Imagine it and rehearse it in your mind, with the body you want. This action will not only change your brain, but rewire your nervous system as well. These changes will then begin to steer your actions automatically. The right choices will become natural instead of being a chore.

Find pictures of these dreams and post them as well. Daydream as much as you can and trace them in your mind often. It is very important to practice this daily and truly *feel it as an actual experience in the present tense*.

Professional athletes practice on and off the field. Some of their most productive practice sessions happen in their minds while lying still. This technique is called mental tracing, and scientists have found some very interesting things about it. When an athlete visualizes a perfect performance in their brain, the nerve impulses actually travel all the way to the muscles and the performance is rehearsed through the nervous system. This makes them more proficient at the given skill without even moving a single muscle fiber.

> "The future belongs to those who believe in the beauty of their dreams."
> —Eleanor Roosevelt

You can't practice these exercises too much. The more you do it, the more skilled you become, and the faster you end up rewiring your brain. Don't be afraid to become obsessive about these thoughts either. Even Obsessive Compulsive Disorder (OCD) is not a bad quality if it is channeled in the right direction. Every successful goal achiever is obsessive to some degree with certain aspects of their life and always with their end goals. Some are even classified as clinical. A few go too far like Howard Hughes, but most are perfectly healthy with a few harmless quirks.

We all have quirks and obsessions. This is a normal part of being human. The key is to direct these anomalies to our advantage and use them as strengths instead of trying to cure them. Obese individuals obsess about food. Instead of trying to "cure" an obsessive personality, it can be retained and simply redirected so they end up obsessing over healthy foods instead.

I'm not trying to get metaphysical or start my own OCD cult here. I'm a proud and committed Christian who believes God is the ultimate power and has the final say in everything. I also believe that He gave us free will and the ability to create our own present situations and shape our own futures. The minds He has given us have more power than most of us realize. These minds will dictate our success or failure. It's His design, and it's your choice.

> *If you cannot see yourself the way you want to be and feel the things you want to do in your mind, the rest of this book will only make you smarter, not fitter.*

Mind's Eye Step Four: Be thankful often.

Put a small sticker on the face of your watch, tie a string on your finger, put a note on your rear view mirror, or anything else you can think of to make you remember to be thankful throughout the day.

Start every day by saying "Thank you." As soon as you wake up, make yourself say it. Even if you feel miserable and can't think of anything to be thankful for, say it anyway and just be thankful that you woke up! Keep saying the words, "Thank you," and pretty soon, even on a Monday morning or after a rough day, you will start to think of things you are thankful for.

This is your subconscious hearing the majority of the messages and acting on them. It is hearing the words, and even though your conscious mind isn't believing it, your subconscious does, and is kicking back thankful thoughts to prove itself right.

Use your reminders to refocus on your goal as well. Be thankful that you have a goal and that you will reach that goal. Be grateful that you are a different person now and celebrate the fact that you have only your future to look to.

Have you ever noticed how different people act on Fridays when compared to Mondays? It is, of course, because they are looking forward to the weekend. Their focus is on their time off in the future and that focus affects their attitude in the present. They are already picturing what they will do and are experiencing that, even though it hasn't happened yet. Focusing on your future self and how that looks and feels will change your present attitude and actions without you even noticing most of these changes.

Being thankful helps create this attitude and perpetuates it. Focusing on what you are grateful for will even change the chemicals in your brain. It raises the levels of the chemicals producing happy feelings and lowers the ones that produce symptoms of depression and anxiety. 60 seconds of grateful thinking can elevate these chemicals in your brain for as long as four hours afterwards!

This chemical change can even turn your hunger cravings around. You can crave sugar less and whole foods more. Your body works according to your attitude and with this action you are literally changing your actual physiology.

Being thankful is yet another way to pull impulses from your negative nerve pathways. Every moment you spend being thankful is another moment causing atrophy of the pathways you want to be rid of. Thoughts of gratitude pull impulses from many negative nerve pathways at the same time so you will atrophy multiple bad habits this way!

Mind's Eye Step Five: Become an optimist.

You may already think you are an optimist and others might even label you as one. It can be true for most aspects in your life, but if you are overweight or out of shape, you are not practicing optimism in those areas. This step will show you how to implement this very important skill and apply it to the part of your being that dictates your shape, body and fitness level.

Practicing steps 1-4 will complement this step, but focusing on the positive side of everything is vital to your success. **This is the most important step**, *but it cannot be achieved without application of the other three.*

This step might take some time to master, so be patient with yourself. Some people get it in a few days; others take more time. It all depends on how much you want to unconsciously hang on to your past and how ingrained it is. If you start to focus on how long it will take, it will certainly take longer. Discouragement will stop your progress completely, so focus only on the little successes along the way.

Practice turning every thought you have into a positive one with conscious choice. You will soon see the patterns that have trapped you where you are, and will enjoy the escape as you master this new skill. You will become a completely new and different person.

It is not only possible to change a negative into a positive, it is imperative if you are to be both mentally and physically well. When you choose positive, happy thoughts, you are much more likely to make healthy choices. Feeling sad or angry leads you to eat poorly and neglect healthy habits. This can then lead to stress and feeling helpless about changing life for the better. The mind and body are so connected that if the mind is unhappy, the body also becomes unwell.

Happiness and optimism is a choice. Abraham Lincoln said, "I have noticed that folks are generally about as happy and they have made up their minds to be." He was very right, and you can make up your mind every day to be happy and become an optimist.

This is of course easier to do when you are rested and not stressed. Almost anyone can be happy on vacation when they are away from work and are getting proper sleep. Even in the hard times however, you can tell yourself you will be happy and will have a good day. Even on a bad day, if you tell yourself over and over that you are happy, pretty soon your subconscious will believe it and make that happen.

Celebrating your successes and focusing on them as progress to your end goal will also give you the patience required. Focusing on the parts of you body that are getting leaner will get you to your goals faster than focusing on the fat that is not coming off, or your "trouble areas." This negative focus will sabotage your progress. Thoughts of despair will certainly keep you there, so every time you are feeling impatient, eject that negative DVD and put on the positive one.

If you think, "I'm going to lose some fat today" you are focusing on the wrong thing and that will make it harder to accomplish. Take your focus off your fat and instead think, "I'm going to become leaner today." It might sound like the same thing, but it really is completely different. Learning this skill and practicing it is vital to your success because you will get better at it, and it will eventually become automatic and part of your personality.

When a tennis player thinks, "Don't miss this serve" or a skier says, "Don't fall" what happens? They do just what they told themselves not to do. If they want success, they need to replace the negative focus with a positive by saying, "I'm going to nail this serve" or, "I can make it down this hill."

> *"Failure is always in the past. It is impossible to fail in the future or even in the present unless you have already decided to."*
> —Anonymous

If you say "Diets never work for me", nothing you try will work. If you say, "I know there is a nutrition plan that will help me achieve my goals" you will find it. When you feel like you are coming down with a cold, don't think, "I really don't want to get sick." That keeps the focus on the cold and will probably make it happen. You can take its power away instead by thinking, "I'm going to stay healthy." Your mind really is that strong!

Habitual negative thoughts actually become wired into your brain like any other thought and the more they are produced, the stronger that wiring becomes. In a relatively short period of time, this wiring becomes an addiction and needs to be fed. The more a nerve pathway is activated, whether positive or negative, the more it craves reactivation.

Chronically negative people have actually become chemically addicted to feeling and thinking negative thoughts. Their negative nerve pathways have been traveled so much, they literally crave these electric impulses. These cravings then cause negative thoughts to be produced so the addiction can be satisfied, and so on, until the downward spiral becomes vicious and very hard to escape from.

Have you ever noticed how tired negative people are, and how energetic positive people are? One major reason for this phenomenon is due to the fact that a negative thought requires about 10 times more energy to produce than a positive thought. Constant negative thoughts sap the energy and drain it from the system.

Positive thoughts actually have a positive energy balance because they require so little energy compared to the result in attitude and hormonal release. This in turn causes an upward spiral, creating more energy and more positive thoughts.

The good news is that even if negative pathways are deeply ingrained, they can be reversed and replaced with positive pathways. Concentrating on the negative pathways and obsessing about not thinking the negative thoughts, will only make them stronger, but ignoring them and replacing them with positive pathways will work without fail.

After a while, the negative pathways don't work any more, and new positive pathways are the ones that are ingrained. You are now addicted to positive thoughts and can enjoy the benefits that follow.

> *A pessimist is one who makes difficulties of his opportunities, and an optimist is one who makes opportunities of his difficulties.*
> —Harry Truman

Most people start a weight loss program and prepare for the "struggle." This is a sure way to fail. You will actually create a struggle by expecting one. If you expect it to take a long time, it will. If you instead focus on the end goal without regard for time or effort, you will reach that goal much faster.

This is also the reason so many people gain the fat back after they lose it. Some even gain back more fat than before, because after they lost the fat, they still focused on keeping it off and avoiding certain foods. The power of their fat and the "bad" foods was still building even after they had reached their goals! Soon, it won and everything went to heck. Even though they did get lean, they never saw themselves that way and then went back to how they did see themselves. The old wiring was still there, and the body simply followed.

Many people have tried to claim the quote, "What you resist, persists." I don't care who coined it, but I'm sure it predates written records because it is a basic truth of life. Resisting something only causes focus on it, and that focus makes it happen.

This applies to nutrition like everything else. If you make a mistake and eat something you shouldn't, forget about it. Beating yourself up over it only ingrains it further in your mind. It is rehearsed again because you are thinking about the mistake, and as far as your nerves are concerned, you just ate it again!

Many people realize the benefits of forgiveness. The release of stress and emotional relief is undeniable. Holding onto anger, resentment, or remorse will put you in a negative downward spiral. This spiral will further ingrain the nerve pathways you are trying to avoid. Forgiving yourself is often harder than forgiving someone else, but it is an important and very necessary step.

If the focus is put on what you should eat, on getting lean, and on staying lean once you get there, you will achieve it and will keep it. This really is the way to finally become the person you always dreamed of. The key is to dream it, believe it, and feel it every day without regard for the negative thoughts and things you are trying to lose or avoid.

Mother Theresa was invited many times to attend anti-war rallies. Each time she declined because she knew how important focusing on the positive was. Her negative nerve pathways were completely atrophied. Her mind was too busy creating positive thoughts, and since positive and negative thoughts cannot occupy the same brain at the same time, she had no time, space or even the ability for the negative ones.

This wonderful woman placed herself in the most horrible areas of our planet and saw some of the most intense suffering imaginable. No matter where she was, she always uplifted those around her and brought a positive result to the situation. Many have marveled at how unaffected she was and how these conditions never dragged her down. Now you know her secret.

> *"I don't attend anti-war rallies. Show me a peace rally and I'll be there."*
> —Mother Theresa

I really can't stress this point too may times, because understanding optimism and positive thinking is the key to your success. Instead of putting the focus on what you don't want to be, you must learn to ignore that and focus on what you do want to be. This is the only way to guaranteed success.

Positive and negative thoughts, decisions and choices are being made by you even though you don't know you are making them. They are a result of your attitude. So many people feel helpless about their weight, and feel that there is nothing they can do, or that they just don't have enough willpower. These thoughts perpetuate themselves until they become true. They become habitual and turn into an attitude that is part of their personality. Their past has become their future.

Leave your fat in the past. That is who you were, not who you are. Tell yourself you are becoming thinner and be thankful for it. Tell yourself every day that you now have a high metabolism. Focus on the picture you chose in step one and visualize yourself that way. Be thankful every day that you are turning into that person.

> *"Optimists are nostalgic about the future."*
> —Unknown

This process takes time. At first your old self will act as saboteur. You may find yourself playing the negative DVDs and feeling discouraged. This is normal, so stay encouraged by that. It is like a tennis match. You will go back and forth and might lose some games, but as long as you win the matches you will end up the champ. The more you practice, the more games and matches you will win. You will defeat your old habits and past history, and replace it with your new future.

You will probably lose weight first in the spots you care the least about. Turn this around and enjoy that success with as much enthusiasm as any other. Fat is fat no matter where it is. Your body will decide where it comes off first, and this is all good. It means your efforts are working and you are on the right track.

When you look in the mirror, concentrate on the areas you feel are the thinnest and be thankful for the parts of you that you do like. When you start to lose weight, focus on those areas only and celebrate them. Pay no regard to the other areas. Ignoring an annoying kid makes him go away. The same rule applies to your "trouble spots." The more you ignore them, the faster they will disappear, and this will be accelerated even more by combining it with focus on your progress areas.

> *"A pessimist complains about the noise when opportunity knocks."*
> —Unknown

I have had clients complain that they are losing their initial weight from the top of their head or even their feet but no where else. I tell them to be very excited because that means it is working just like it should. They are losing fat! I then tell them that if they only focus on the fat not coming off a certain spot, it never will. They will unconsciously keep it from happening with little actions they don't even know they are doing. If they focus instead on getting leaner, and celebrate the areas where that is happening with no regard for what area that is, they will eventually lean out in their "trouble spots" as well.

Fat will probably come off of your extremities first because that is the most inefficient place for your body to carry it. Your body knows that storing fat around your center of gravity is the easiest place to carry it. Putting it on your hands or feet however, is less efficient because they move more and swing around, so fat will be gained there last and come off there first.

When you walk up a staircase, you can only see the flight you are on, but you can climb a multi-story building and get to the top stair without seeing it until the last flight. On the other hand, some staircases are built so you can see all the way up, but even if they are shorter, they seem harder to climb because you are focusing on how far you have to go.

I often run stairs in a 63 floor building in downtown Seattle. I'm glad I can only see one flight at a time, because if I could see all the way to the top, I would really have to concentrate on not psyching myself out. One flight at a time is mentally much easier to grasp, and after about 7 minutes, I'm at the top floor.

Losing fat from the top of your head first is fantastic. So what if no one but you can notice. It's like the set of stairs in front of you that you can see. When you keep going, there will be another flight just around the corner that might represent fat lost from the back of your heels and so on until you reach the top stair and find the fat is gone from every area you wanted.

> *"Take the first step in faith. You don't have to see the whole staircase, just take the first step."*
> —Martin Luther King Jr.

We all know "lucky" people. They are no luckier than you. They just feel that way and know how to spot opportunity better because of it. A study was done by a psychologist to test the difference between "lucky" people and those who labeled themselves "unlucky." He printed a booklet with 30 pictures in it, along with some text and instructions at the beginning which read "Find out how many pictures are in this book and report your results back to me."

On page three he put in bold letters, right in the middle paragraph, "There are 30 pictures. Stop counting now." The "lucky" people saw this and stopped counting. The "unlucky" people missed it and kept counting. They never saw the opportunity even though it was obvious.

One of my professors in college was a world class Olympic coach. He taught many of the athletes who are now household names, and some of the most famous ones had "lucky socks" or a "lucky shirt." Instead of telling them that superstitions are silly, he would provide a combination lock safe for the athletes to store those items, and would then sleep in front of the safe to add another perceived level of security. He knew the items weren't lucky, but because the athletes believed they were, he knew they would perform better with them. He chose to reinforce the superstition and make it more powerful, instead of trying to convince the athletes of reality.

Lucky charms aren't really lucky. It's our belief in them that makes us act lucky and open our eyes to the opportunities available. Placebo drugs have been found in many cases to be even more effective than real medicine. In fact, almost half of the doctors admit to prescribing placebos to their patients. You probably have received a placebo and chances are, it worked as well or better than a real drug. Your attitude really is that powerful, and with a little practice, your mind can produce this power.

As you change your thinking, you will also change those around you. Birds of a feather really do flock together. If you find yourself surrounded by people with lots of problems, it's probably the way you think of your own life. As you become an optimist, you will find yourself attracting these people to you, and you to them. Pretty soon you will have a whole new set of friends that help you and lift you up, and your old friends who used to drag you down will want in on the secret you have discovered.

Have you ever looked in an old school yearbook and found that many of the "popular" kids were actually pretty funny looking? Everyone thought that person was good looking back then but, that's only because they were confident on the inside. They felt good looking regardless of whether they were or not, and everyone else believed it.

Another good example of this can be found among our current pop culture. Most of our top rock stars are either ugly as sin, or surprisingly average looking, yet millions see them as simply drop-dead gorgeous. If half of them were found walking on the street with no fame or fortune, they would be just another average looking person, turning no heads at all.

Every great man or woman in history has been an optimist. Good things happened to them because they expected them to. We are all offered the same amount of opportunities in life. The optimists just know how to see them better.

"No pessimist ever discovered the secret of the stars, or sailed to an uncharted land, or opened a new doorway to the human spirit."
—Helen Keller

Pessimists are typically the way they are because of being hurt at some point or developing the habit over time from repeated pain. Being a pessimist might feel safer but it's not. It is a sure way to bring more misfortune and hurt upon yourself. Pessimists feel safer because they are either constantly being proven right or pleasantly surprised. This is just a smoke screen however, because expecting the worst not only makes it happen, but it also clouds your vision against seeing the best things life has to offer.

Some of the most prosperous people in the world have had the toughest lives. We all have a sob story, and we all have accumulated baggage. To be successful at your goals is to leave that behind and form the attitude for success. It's what we do now, and from now on that makes average people great.

As you play these positive mental DVD's to yourself, you will become this person, and will attract the same kind of people to yourself. This will turn into an upward spiral perpetuating itself and help you reach your goals even faster. The downward spirals of your past have been forgotten, have atrophied, and have lost their power. They might be who you were, but are no longer who you are or will be in the future.

Sir Thomas Brown wrote in 1642, "I am the happiest man alive. I have that in me that can convert poverty to riches, adversity to prosperity, and I am more invulnerable than Achilles." He certainly looked at the positive side of things and found success very easily as a result.

> "Whether you think you can or you can't,
> either way you are right"
> —Henry Ford

CHAPTER THREE

CRACKING THE "FIT" CODE

What is "fit" anyway? This is the most important question of all because if you don't know the answer, you may never be satisfied with your own fitness, and will be endlessly chasing an elusive "rainbow." A very talented writer from the Seattle Times, asked me this question recently for one of his articles, and it forced me to put into writing some deeply rooted thoughts I have developed over the years from working with so many different kinds of people.

If you ask a traditional trainer this question, they will probably try to spew things like fitness formulas and V02 max norms, but what it really comes down to is the fact that the definition of "fit" is very individual and subjective.

I have trained plenty of people who might not slide into the clinical definition of "fit" but feel like they are, and are happy and content with their level of fitness. Then there are others who score above the 90th percentile in the "norms" but feel like they are still pathetically out of shape. I would classify the first person as more "fit" because they believe in themselves more and have the confidence that seeps outward to be seen by others.

The more narcissistic someone is, the less likely they will be to become fit in their own opinion. Unfortunately, these arc the kinds of people that are drawn to the fitness industry. The cover models for fitness and bodybuilding magazines are usually more critical of themselves than "normal" people outside the industry. They are chasing a rainbow they will never reach. Contentment will always elude them.

The professional fitness competitors and bodybuilders often use the terms "ripped" or "shredded" to define their fitness. These terms relate to the subcutaneous body fat, otherwise known as the fat under the skin. 10% body fat is considered "defined", 8% is "cut", 5% is "ripped", and 3% is "shredded." This varies slightly between people, but even this rating has very little to do with being fit. There are plenty of people who have 5% body fat but are very out of shape or have an eating disorder.

There are plenty of bodybuilders who look "shredded" and indeed come out around 3% body fat when measured with skinfold calipers, but are in fact 12-18% body fat when the internal fat is measured with full-body measurement equipment. This huge discrepancy is due to the excessive visceral fat that stores internally around their organs, built up from use of illegal anabolic drugs and hormones. This is why you won't find a professional bodybuilder who is willing to submit themselves for testing methods outside of skinfold calipers.

Professional bodybuilders and most professional fitness competitors must take these illegal anabolic drugs to compete at the world class level. Because of the personality types that are drawn to this sport, many other unhealthy habits often extend beyond the use of drugs.

These "athletes" are the least healthy participants of any sport or game in existence, despite the fact that they are regarded by some as the healthiest "looking" people. They may look fit on the outside, but they are a broken down mess on the inside, and die prematurely from cancer, organ failure or some other drug related cause. Many bodybuilders put themselves on the organ transplant lists before they even have symptoms because they know that what they are doing is surely killing them! It is a true shame that these are the people society (especially kids) look up to as the picture of "fit!"

Most people get into fitness because they don't like themselves. They think becoming fit will solve this problem, and guess what? It doesn't. The vast majority within the fitness industry have a lower self image than those on the outside! Sure, they look fit, but it didn't help like they thought it would. Then they push harder and further, and get into steroids and drugs chasing after that moving finish line, and end up much unhealthier than they were before.

"Fit" is a very broad spectrum and is more of a bell curve. Most of the cover models on fitness magazines are not "fit" at all. They may be "skinny" but their muscle mass is relatively low and their lifestyle is probably not the healthiest either.

I place morbidly obese individuals as far away from the middle of the bell curve as the professional bodybuilders. This is another unhealthy and certainly unfit population who are physical time bombs winding down fast. Morbidly obese individuals have about the same lifespan as the pro bodybuilders, and almost the same rate of cancer and organ failure as well.

Also sitting to the side of the bell curve are the people who are too skinny and may suffer from eating disorders. Either side of the curve is full of people with psychological issues they need to get worked out before they can make the move to become "fit." Their brain wiring is so ingrained, it really is a strong addiction. Anyone can reverse and rewire their brains however, so no one should despair!

"Fit" to me are the people in the middle of the bell curve. Some may be 20 lbs. overweight, but are content with who they are and can perform in sports and activities to their satisfaction. Others may be naturally "skinny" and technically underweight, but eat very healthy and take good care of themselves.

If you like who you are, you will take good care of yourself, and "fit" will be a priority often happening as a byproduct of a clean and active lifestyle. It is an internal thing as well as external. Learning to like yourself and how to realize contentment is the most important step in becoming "fit." Practicing the techniques in section one toward this end is the fastest way to get there, and the only way to ensure that it is permanent.

Muscle mass is another important factor in being fit. To be fit in a well rounded way, you need muscle to provide you with a high metabolism and the physical strength and endurance necessary for the activities you want to enjoy. Older people become less fit with age mainly because they slow down and lose muscle. Jack LaLanne is in his 90's now and still runs circles around most people in their 20's.

While obese individuals are never physically fit, overweight people can be. They can do activities and enjoy sports and recreation thoroughly. They can be attractive physically as well. I would much rather see someone with muscle and some extra fat on them than the "skinny" cover model with little muscle.

While "fit" is a subjective definition (as it should be), it is often redefined unnecessarily by those who don't have the right mindset for it. There is a term I like to use called "Contentment Deficit Disorder" (CDD) and this condition exists with most Americans (and with people in other prosperous countries).

Most of those with CDD have trouble being content with themselves and their situation. When a person with CDD achieves a preset fitness goal, it suddenly isn't good enough any more, so they set another one and "move their finish line." This pattern is often repeated until they give up out of frustration and then backslide, ending up worse off than where they started. They forgot they flew by their original goal without acknowledging their success. People do this with other things in their lives as well like spouses, money, houses, jobs, and more.

This type of affliction will keep anyone from being fit. To be truly fit you must learn to be content with your accomplishments and then if more "fit" comes along, it's just a bonus. I know this firsthand because I have reached my goals, am content with how I look, and can physically do anything I desire, so I am fully content staying where I am now. This is really the last and most important step to becoming "fit."

Most people think that contentment comes from getting what we want. True contentment however, is *wanting what we get*. The single most important key to achieving fitness is mastering contentment. Setting short and long term goals is of course important, but what is most important is being content when you reach them.

If you pass up your short term goals without recognizing them and taking time to celebrate them, they will become less meaningful. If you keep moving your finish line like most people do, you will never be happy with your results, and fitness will merely be a continual frustration.

CHAPTER FOUR

CRACKING YOUR CALORIE CODE

How would you like to throw calorie counting out the window, or eat as much as you want of certain foods without gaining fat? New breakthroughs in nutrition research and human physiology have discovered that not all calories are created equal, and certain foods will actually make you lose more fat the more you eat them!

Dieticians and nutritionists have long preached the "calorie in—calorie out" theory. This theory is still a theory, because it hasn't been proven with science. In fact, there is more scientific evidence against the theory than for it, and the studies that seem to support it are flawed or misinterpreted.

We aren't machines that can be described by a formula or predicted with math. The body is smarter than we give it credit for. Gorging on a big Thanksgiving dinner doesn't have proportionate weight gains like the theory would have you assume, because of the metabolism increase from overfeeding. Feces are very calorie dense, but dieticians seem to completely ignore this basic bodily function, and don't count those calories out even though they are being flushed down the toilet and not absorbed by the body at all.

Science has discovered that our physiology and metabolism are much too complex and dynamic to be defined by general calculations. Because of this new understanding, scientists have recently been working feverishly to crack the code and figure out what does work, and more importantly, why.

We have all been taught that each gram of protein or carbohydrate holds four calories, each gram of fat holds 9 calories, and each gram of alcohol holds 7 calories. This is true inside a beaker, but inside your body it is a different story, and inside someone else's body it's yet another story.

Even though protein and carbs both contribute 4 calories per gram, they have vastly different effects on your metabolism. A gram of lean protein in the form of meat, raises your metabolism significantly for a relatively long period of time for an overall positive metabolic effect. A gram of carbs in the form of sugar on the other hand, raises your metabolism for a very short time and then crashes it, with a resulting overall negative metabolic effect.

A gram of fat has very little effect on metabolic elevation so the net effect is usually negative, but there are different kinds of fat that have different effects as well. Alcohol always lowers your metabolism in every case, so the effects of this type of calorie are detrimental to your metabolism without any exceptions.

Protein is the highest metabolic type of calorie, and meat is always the best source of protein. Organic meat is the best choice for poultry, and wild fish is the best seafood. Organic grass-fed beef is more than twice as good as plain organic beef for fat burning benefits because of the type of fat it contains. The calories are all the same between these different forms of protein, but the effects on your metabolism are very different.

Whey sources are also a high quality protein as long as your digestive system can handle milk products. Whey protein shakes are a quick and easy way to get protein without the carbs and fat, and taken right before bed, can even raise your growth hormone levels during the night.

Cottage cheese is another good night time protein source because it has a built-in time release mechanism since it takes so much more time to break down than other dairy sources. This time release feature can keep your metabolism elevated during the night for increased fat burning and even spare some muscle breakdown.

Whey protein and cottage cheese protein both hold 4 calories per gram, but because they are made up of very different kinds of protein, they have very different effects on your metabolism. They both have positive metabolic effects, but for different reasons and provide different fat burn rates.

You will sometimes see food labels list carbohydrates with one number and then "impact carbs" or "net carbs" with another number. These terms represents the actual number of carbs that have an impact on your calorie level. A gram of fiber is also a gram of carbohydrate, but because of fiber's effects, it can be subtracted from the total carbohydrate count so it cancels itself out. My favorite salsa has 3 grams of carbs per serving and 2 grams of fiber so the impact on my system is 1 carb.

Other types of carbs can lower the overall impact number as well. Sugar alcohols (sorbitol, maltitol, and glycerol), are the main carb source found in low carb foods. The labeling laws require food manufacturers to list the total carbs regardless of impact, so when foods contain non-impact carbs, they list their own "real" carbs separately. I'm not a big fan of sugar alcohols, so my recommendation is to reduce your carb count through natural fiber instead.

Fat always holds 9 calories per gram, but not all fat stores the same way and certain types of fat actually help you burn fat off your body. In fact, too little fat can even prevent you from burning body fat. Saturated fat works different in your body than unsaturated fat. Omega 3 oils provide benefits that omega 6 oils cancel out with the wrong balance between the two, but both are needed in the right proportions.

I know this all sounds confusing, and you really don't have to learn all the details of ratios and calorie differences. It is helpful however, to have a general understanding of how it all works and the flaws with conventional nutrition "wisdom." This book will show you how to make this whole process easy, so hang in there and the good news will sink in!

Different fats end up being stored in different places in the body. Saturated fat tends to store in your "trouble spots" as well as your internal blood vessels, often causing cardiovascular disease. Unsaturated fat still stores just as well in your "trouble spots", but not as well in your blood vessels, so it is generally thought of as more healthy.

Omega 3 fats also store in your "trouble spots" like any other fat, but they contribute to brain health as a side benefit. Omega 6 fats are necessary as well, but too much of them combined with too little Omega 3 will create an imbalance pushing out Omega 3 and cancelling the positive brain benefits. I emphasize this particular imbalance because there is so much soy present in processed foods, that we typically get too much Omega 6 and not enough Omega 3 fats.

Some fats are manufactured by our own body, but some can only be found in food. These fats are called essential fatty acids. Certain vitamins are also considered essential, while others are made by your body.

Alcohol is the final major macronutrient. It gives 7 calories per gram, and always in every case, slows your metabolism and makes you store fat. Your fat burning is completely stopped, and your fat storage is turned on while your body is processing it.

Drinks with higher alcohol content will of course have a worse metabolic effect, but drinks with high carbs and sugars will provide a poor calorie combination as well. Alcohol carbs can be thought of the same as fat carbs.

I could talk about all the different kinds of protein, carbs, fats, alcohols, and vitamins, but those topics could fill another book, and would just be too confusing anyway. It really is simpler than anyone realizes, and the advice found in this book will give you the shortcuts you are looking for.

Most people have heard that if they burn 3500 calories more than they take in, they will lose one pound. If that's the case then why does that so often fail? Why do some seem to lose more than a pound from burning less than 3500 calories and others lose little to nothing for vast amounts of effort?

No one should be concerned with losing body weight as much as losing fat weight. A pound of fat actually holds more than 4,000 calories, and a pound of muscle less than 2,000 calories. A pound of water can be lost easier than fat or muscle and it has no calories at all. If you burn 3,500 extra calories with exercise, the energy spent will never come exclusively from fat stores anyway. It will always be a mixture of water, fat, carbs, and sometimes muscle.

How you exercise makes all the difference in the world with your burn mixture. There will be no math required or formulas to learn in this book because it is all about when, how, and what, when it comes to nutrition and exercise. The following calculations are included only to prove my point of how wrong traditional formulas are, and how the very concept is completely outdated.

I weigh 170 pounds, so I burn about 550 calories in an hour of regular cardio exercise at the best fat burning intensity. Since I would burn 150 calories doing nothing in that time anyway, my extra calories burned comes to 400.

Since even the most ideal "fat burning zone" cardio burns about 50 percent calories from fat and 50 percent from carbs, I will burn about 200 more fat calories than if I had done nothing at all, right? Wrong, because if I had done nothing, my fuel mixture would have been about 75 percent from fat (since I am a primary fat burner) so I would have burned about 113 calories from fat just lying around. This brings my net fat burning benefit to a whopping 87 calories for my hour of cardio sweat.

By these calculations, 87 fat calories equals about 10 grams of fat, which equals about a third of an ounce. To lose a pound of fat simply through the exercise time itself, I would need to work out for almost 50 hours. I don't know anyone who would put this kind of effort into that small of a payout!

The good news is that exercise does give you a heightened metabolism after you have completed the activity. Regular cardio is about a one-to-one ratio, meaning if you work out for an hour, your metabolism will stay elevated for another hour after you are done. This post-exercise metabolic elevation mixture is a much higher fat fuel burn ratio than the exercise itself, so more fat is burned than is represented in the exercise time alone.

After all this is factored in, the time required to burn a pound of fat is only reduced to about 20 hours of cardio. This still isn't fast enough to keep most people motivated. I don't even have the patience for those diminished returns. I certainly don't have that kind of attention span.

The good news is that high intensity exercise has a drastically different fat burning result, and takes much less time. A 20 minute high intensity session may burn less calories than the hour long regular cardio during the exercise time itself, and only 20 percent of the calories might come from fat during that 20 minute workout, but the after effects last three to four hours with an unusually higher fat burning rate! This puts the overall fat loss higher with the 20 minute high intensity cardio for that day, than the hour long regular cardio did by a long shot.

The bottom line however, is the fact that the fastest way to lose fat is through proper nutrition. This involves choosing the types of calories and forgetting about the amount of calories. I could eat 2,000 calories a day of the wrong food and gain fat and lose muscle simultaneously. I could also eat 4,000 calories of the right food and lose fat while gaining muscle. No one can get fatter eating white meat and broccoli no matter what the amount, but anyone can gain fat eating Halloween candy and holiday carbs, even in small amounts.

Scientists have found that the timing of food is crucial. Dieticians will tell you it's still about the number of calories no matter when you eat them. If you want to test this theory yourself, just try fasting all day and then eat all your calories in ice cream right before you go to bed and see what happens!

I just counseled a woman who lost 5 pounds of fat in 3 weeks from one small change in her nutrition habits. All she did was take the banana out of her morning protein shake. In 3 weeks, this only represented a total calorie reduction of 3000 calories less than before, but instead of losing less than 1 pound over that 3 weeks like a dietician would have predicted, she lost more than five times that amount. It was the kind of calorie and the timing of that calorie that made all the difference and recent research sheds some light on why.

Debra was simply cutting her fat burning window short with the type of sugar found in the banana. If we sleep a full night without any midnight snacks, we all wake up in our highest fat burning state. Because we have been fasting all night, we have moved into our fat burning zone by the time we wake up. Certain types of calories will cause this to shut down and others will let it continue so we can stretch this fat burning window further into the day.

Her protein shake in the morning was a good idea. Because we are also typically starting our muscle burning state in the morning as well, protein will shut that down. Interrupting the muscle burning state is a good thing because you will want to keep that tissue. Fat burning however, is a different story because most of us want to lose as much fat as we can.

While the protein was effectively shutting down the muscle burning process, the banana was shutting down the fat burning process by increasing the insulin and providing carbs for a fuel source to replace the fat fuel source. Taking the banana out of the protein shake allowed her body to extend the fat burning window further into the day, and shut down the muscle burning process.

The typical American diet is very high in carbs, so when most Americans go to sleep, blood glucose is used for energy first. About 2 hour's worth is typically available in the blood. When this is used up, the body takes more out of the liver. About 3 hour's worth is available there. When both of these stores are used up, fat has to kick in as the primary fuel source. This fat burn zone goes on for about 2 hours until the metabolism starts to slow down and protein begins to be used. This is when muscle burning begins.

You can see how a dinner low in carbs and high in protein will start your fat burning zone earlier. You will run out sooner and will be forced into the fat burning zone sooner. The protein you ate for dinner will also spare your muscle by being available to be burned as fuel instead of having to be cannibalized from your muscle tissue.

A breakfast also high in protein and low in carbs will stretch that window on the other end and shut down any muscle burning that might have started. You can burn 10 times the amount of fat you otherwise would have, by just changing your breakfast and dinner habits!

Sumo wrestlers have found through hundreds of years of experience that the best way to get fat in the shortest time is to fast all day and then gorge on carbs and fat at night. Unfortunately, most of us eat this way too. We get up too late to eat breakfast or just settle for coffee and a donut. The caffeine and sugar put us into an energy crash by lunch time, so we seek out more sugar to pick us back up. The calories themselves are relatively low because we are too busy at work to eat much volume. By the time we get home we are famished, and now that we have the time, we eat . . . . and eat . . . and eat. The types of food are also perfect to ensure fat storing all night long. No wonder we have so may more sumo candidates in this country than Japan!

I said it before and I'll say it again: All calories are certainly not created equal (as an outdated dietician would have you believe). It's not the type of calorie that is the issue, or even the amount of calories. It's the combination of certain calories that will make you fat. Fat by itself won't make you gain fat. Carbs by themselves won't either. It's the combination of the two that will add to your waistline. Certain carbs and fast sugars will spike your insulin and put you in a "storing mode." This mode will make your body absorb all types of macronutrients (protein, carbs and fat) at a faster rate.

This is good if you are eating protein with fast carbs, but bad if you are eating fast carbs with fat. It's not the rice or potatoes that will increase your belt size. It's those foods with the toppings, butter, and other fatty ingredients that will cause the problems.

When your pancreas releases insulin, your body immediately inhibits your fat burning hormone called hormone-sensitive lipase (HSL). This hormone's job is to release fat into your bloodstream to be burned off as it is used for fuel. When HSL is inhibited through elevated insulin, your body will run on amino acids from your muscles and carbohydrates for its fuel source instead of fat.

Being in this state causes you to be unusually hungry, which further feeds this vicious cycle. The key is to keep your insulin levels low so your HSL stays high and is able to facilitate your fat burning state all day and night.

The donut is the best example of the wrong combinations of macronutrients and the perfect food for spiking your insulin. Being made of dough, sugar and fat and in the perfect wrong proportions, make this the ultimate fat storing tool. The donut starts as simple starchy dough. This in itself would be enough to raise insulin levels to the fat storing mode, but it doesn't stop there. The next stage is the 360 degree vegetable oil that cooks the donuts just long enough to sear in sufficient amounts of fat for optimum storage in your cells.

The cooking process also alters the dough enough to introduce cancer cells in your system. The sugar coating at the end of the process is about twice that required to spike your insulin levels, so fat storage is guaranteed while the fat burning system is almost completely shut down. If you eat the jelly filled variety, then you get sugar on the inside as well as the outside. If you were to create the perfect fat increasing food, it would be the donut.

Krispy Kreme, the inventor of the uniform donut and automated donut machine, has the capability to produce 7.5 billion donuts per year. In about 22 seconds, Krispy Kreme stores together can produce enough donuts to make a stack higher than the Empire State Building.

If I were to develop the ideal fat gaining program for a Sumo wrestler, I would start him each day at Krispy Kreme with donuts and a coffee. Then I'd have him sit around all day at a computer or in front of a TV until dinner. His dinner would be pasta and wine, with some more donuts and ice cream for desert. This macronutrient ratio and timing is not too far off the typical American's daily habits, so it's no wonder we are so fat!

Conventional wisdom tells us to eat fewer calories and exercise more. I have talked to many frustrated people who are already doing this but are only going backwards as a result. When I get them to exercise less and eat more, they lose weight like crazy! It's all in *how* you exercise, *what* you eat and *when* you eat it that makes the difference.

Calories are not the enemy. In fact, I didn't get as lean as I am now until I increased my calorie level from 2500 per day to 4000 per day. It is the types of calories I eat and the kinds of food I consume that keep me at or below a steady 7% body fat level all year around.

My daily nutrition habits keep me in a fat burning mode all day and all night. Since I am never hungry in the morning because of my genetic type, I drink a protein shake to start my day. I use natural chocolate whey protein sweetened with Stevia and mixed with organic vanilla soy milk. I use two scoops of whey powder and a whole quart of soy milk. This takes about 2 hours for me to drink down and contains about 70 grams of protein, 40 grams of carbs, and 15 grams of fat for a total of 575 calories.

This breakfast is enough to revive my metabolism from the nighttime decline but since I drink it over the course of a couple hours, and the carbs are slow absorbing, my insulin never has a chance to spike. This causes the fat to be burned and used for energy instead of stored. Since my body is looking for protein in the morning, it will absorb that without the need of assistance from insulin.

The quart of soy milk in the morning also rehydrates me so I can get back to where I left off the night before. I am usually two pounds lighter when I wake up than when I went to bed. This is almost exclusively due to the water vapor I exhaled during sleep. Two pounds is a quart, so drinking my shake in the morning gets me back to where I need to be pretty fast.

Since it is clean organic soy milk, it is very absorbable (unlike coffee, which has a negative hydration effect).

My next meal is whenever my hunger gets to a 7 on a scale of 1-10. This is usually between 11am-1pm. Lunch consists of a mixture of grass-fed ground beef, organic broccoli, organic spinach, and organic egg whites. I cook it the night before and bring it with me to work in Tupperware. I eat that until I am at a 4 on the 1-10 hunger scale and stop. Within a half an hour I am down to a 1-2 on the hunger scale and feel completely satisfied.

I repeat this cycle for the rest of the work day and eat whenever I am at a 7 and stop at a 4. By the time I get home, I have polished off 2-3 pounds of ground grass-fed beef, a pound of broccoli, and a pound of spinach, for a new daily subtotal of about 3000 calories. I have also sipped on pure, filtered water constantly through the day, to the tune of about two quarts.

When I get home I broil another pound of broccoli and cook some other type of meat (usually salmon) on my Foreman grill. Sometimes I will have some organic rice chips with organic bean dip for an extra treat if I am in the mood for some crunchies. I will drink another quart of filtered water with a packet of EmergenC for flavor and a dash of Stevia. I finish the day by eating about 8 ounces of lowfat cottage cheese for a bedtime snack.

This brings my daily total to a gallon of liquid, about 4,000 calories, and plenty of protein to stoke my metabolism. I never get hungry, my energy is always optimal, and my cravings are only for the proper foods.

With these habits, most people would call me a fanatic, but I certainly don't feel like one. It's easy now, and my body craves these things. When I do go out with friends or feast with the family on Thanksgiving, my metabolism can handle it and simply adjusts up to burn it all off because of my new and firm metabolic set point.

No one will reach these kinds of habits overnight and if you expect to immediately start eating this way, you will be disappointed and end in frustration and failure. It took me time to get to this point and the same will be for you. Now that I am there however, and because I have followed the principles and techniques in this book, I have no more struggles. My cravings are only for the best foods and if I eat processed foods now, I really feel the negative effects because I am so detoxified. Knowing those effects will result are another way my body is now repulsed by the very thought of those foods.

My metabolic readings on any machine I have used always come in between 1900-2200 calories a day for a basal metabolic rate, but I am eating twice that and staying extremely lean. In fact, I sometimes dip down below

6% body fat and then have to eat peanut butter sandwiches to get my fat level back up! I am never battling to keep my fat down like everyone else. It's only the other way if anything.

Many people attribute my lean levels to the fact that I work at a gym every day. They say, "If I worked at a gym full time, I'd probably look like you too." Exercise isn't the main explanation for my low body fat however. I now do strength training once a week for 20 minutes and cardio 2-3 times a week for 8 minutes per session. On a very active week when I have lots of time to work out, I still train less than an hour TOTAL for the whole week, including cardio and weights.

My job is actually fairly sedentary because as the owner of three gyms, I have lots of administrative things to do and find myself sitting down at a desk or computer most of the day or counseling clients. I am in fact the most sedentary I have ever been in my life.

I used to have to work at staying below 10% body fat. I exercised much more and ate much less than I do now and found it a constant struggle to stay lean. I would look in the mirror and see all the fat areas I wanted to lose and concentrated on those. Everything turned around however, as soon as I changed my mind set, exercise habits, and nutrition practices.

Now when I look in the mirror, I celebrate how lean I am. I eat whenever I am hungry and don't even think about how much or when I am eating. My exercise routine takes much less time and frees me up to do the things I love, like spend more time with my family and counsel clients.

CRACKING THE HOLIDAY CALORIE CODE

Have you ever wondered why grocery stores put out their Halloween candy early in September? I'll bet you know the answer. They count on the fact that we will rationalize buying it by telling ourselves it will be for the trick-or-treaters, saying something like, "Since I'm here, I'd better get that candy now so I won't have to worry about it later when it's too late and they have run out."

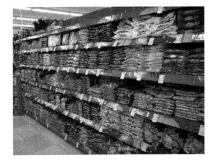

We all know good and well they won't run out and in fact, will still have so much left over they will mark it down "50% off" after Halloween. This of course is another marketing ploy to get us to buy some for "the holidays" or even, "next Halloween."

So we give in to the marketing and buy our bag of candy in September. Some of us even go so far as to actually put it out in a bowl by the door to convince ourselves our intentions were pure. Five or six bowls later, Halloween rolls around and by then, the average American has spent more than $15 on Halloween candy, but less than $3 of that will be given out to the kiddies. When the dust has finally settled each year, America has spent over $1 billion on Halloween candy alone!

While this is, of course, a personal atrocity, the worst ramifications of this habit occur in your own brain. You have started an avalanche in the way your neurons work, and if not interrupted; it will guarantee another year of cyclic holiday weight gain (always successful), followed by the New Year's resolution of weight loss (rarely successful).

The holiday calorie code is a vicious cycle that seems to repeat itself no matter what we do to prevent it. Willpower doesn't seem to be the issue, because it happens to many people with plenty of that to spare. In order to break this cycle we must first understand our own brains and how they work.

What we are doing without realizing it, is brainwashing ourselves into this holiday cycle. Starting in September, we gear up the nerves in our brain by firing the synapses that crave these treats. The brain doesn't know the difference between eating a certain food and thinking about a certain food. It's the same nerve pathway being traveled either way.

Every time we travel a nerve pathway, it gets deeper and stronger. That's how athletes improve with practice and also how cravings and 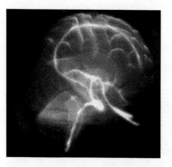 addictions become ingrained. It all starts when we go in the store and see the candy (nerve pathway activation #1). Then we buy the candy (same nerve pathway activation, but now it's being traveled a second time). Then we caress the candy and maybe even give it a quick hug when we take it out of the shopping bag at home (third nerve activation for that pathway). Then we open the bag and smell the sugar (activation #4). Then we open the first candy bar and hear the familiar crackle of the wrapper (activation #5). Then we eat the candy, but of course we have to sample the other ones because we bought the variety pack (activations #6-23). Some of you reading this will notice your mouth is watering already.

By this time, we might as well take that candy and "get a room" because the public display of affection is too much to bear, even though we are alone in our homes and the dog is the only one watching.

Next, you limit yourself to only one piece at a time so you don't get "carried away" and won't "run out" for the "trick-or-treaters" you "bought the candy for." Piece by piece, the bowl empties out. You couldn't possibly have eaten that much so fast! You are sure it is the kids eating too much or the spouse is just being a pig. Heck, the dog probably has been jumping up and sneaking singles too. He's really smart—just eating one at a time so you won't notice, and then making sure his whiskers are wiped off to hide the evidence. Ah hah! That's where those mystery spots in the carpet are coming from! It's the darn dog cleaning off his whiskers!

Now you are mad because everyone else gobbled up the candy you bought for the kiddies! How could they? Well, this time you get two bags to refill the bowl so there will surely be enough left when Halloween rolls around in seven weeks. That bowl disappears too and all along the way, whether you are eating it consciously or automatically, you are making your cravings stronger. Even thinking about it when you are away from the bowl makes the cravings more ingrained since the brain doesn't know the difference between eating it and thinking about it.

Next you decide to bring the candy to the office because everyone else in your house has obviously lost control. Surely your friends at work will be much more considerate than your family, and since dogs aren't allowed, you can check that one off the list too. To your surprise however, the candy disappears faster than ever. How could this be, since you are positive you are eating way less than you did at home? Everyone else denies it and to your dismay, you discover you are now surrounded by bunch of liars you previously thought you could trust!

By the time Halloween does finally come, you have effectively brainwashed yourself into being a sugar junkie. A recent study compared cocaine craving to sugar craving, and guess which one won? The sugar craving was actually hardest to give up! Next comes Thanksgiving and all the candy, cranberry sauce, drinks, and desserts with it. Then Christmas, with the cookies, gingerbread, frosting, and so on.

By this time our stomach's capacity has been stretched so it can accommodate more food. It takes almost 30% more food to get the same sensation of "fullness" than it did before the holidays! Couple this with a little wine which increases the appetite (especially for carbs and fat), and the fact that alcohol specifically attacks the fat burning metabolism, and it's a wonder we don't all look like Jiminy Glick by year's end!

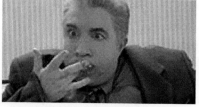

Let's not even go into the days in between the actual holidays. The nibbling and grazing that occurs to satisfy these addictions is phenomenal—especially the fact that most of it is unconscious. Our brainwashing has been so effective; we don't even know what we are eating any more!

Finally it's time for the New Year parties. We are starting to feel bad about the weight we've put on. But it's OK because we wear long pants and coats in the winter to cover it all up. We will worry about the weight problem in January after our one last hurrah on New Year's Eve! This New Year's resolution will be SERIOUS, and the weight will certainly come off this time! Yeah, right.

When it is time to start your New Year's "diet", you are already fighting an uphill battle. You now have addictions and cravings formed with deep rooted nerve pathways that are so hard to break, that by the end of January you have given up. This is mainly because now that you aren't eating the sugar any more, you are thinking about those foods five times more often than you thought about them *and* ate them before the diet. Guess what this is doing? Yep, your cravings are getting even worse despite the fact you aren't eating those things at all. That's why you rebound so much when you go off the diet!

You have now become addicted to your addictions. Your brain craves these addictive nerve pathways and yearns to feed them and activate them. You think you feel better when you feed your addictions but when you are over them and look back, you realize how horrible those habits made you feel.

So now that you understand the holiday calorie code, how do you crack it? By using the brainwashing process to help you instead of hurt you. Thinking of alternatives to the sugar foods when those thoughts come into your brain stops the negative impulses from carving deeper channels and instead activates the impulses you want to become stronger.

This thought-switching process gets easier with practice and prevents the holiday brainwash. You can also plan ahead each day and bring some cut up fruit to replace the candy. Drink a glass of water when an urge hits. Have some frozen blueberries instead of those special edition holiday colored M&M's. If you do have a cookie or piece of candy, don't have a second. Check that one off the list so that particular pathway won't be traveled again.

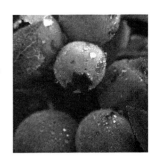

Simply switching your thoughts can be enough to reverse the negative brainwash. Tell yourself every morning that you will make healthy choices that day. Tell yourself this will be your fittest holiday season. Say this out loud in the mirror so you activate multiple positive pathways and ingrain them deeper with each practice.

Even if this only partially works and you gain just half the weight you normally do, getting it off with your resolution will be more than twice as fast as before because you aren't fighting the uphill battle of hundreds of deep and ingrained pathways to overcome and reverse! What have you got to lose? Or more importantly, think about what you have NOT got to gain!

There is hope for everyone, and the only thing you can do to ensure your failure is *the same thing you have always done*. Repeating these same failures year after year only convinces your brain that it is hopeless and makes failure more likely each year. It's time to try something truly different this year that actually works!

CHAPTER FIVE

CRACKING THE OVEREATING CODE

Overeating is more than just a bad habit or willpower issue. It can be a very real physical addiction. Overeating releases certain hormones and chemicals in the brain and body that cause chain reactions which can create and feed addictions. Such addictions can be strong and extremely hard to break.

Certain foods can trigger these addictions and certain ingredients can contribute as well. As mentioned previously, junk food manufacturers know very well which ingredients encourage addictions and they include them in their foods for that purpose.

We also eat for emotional reasons. We medicate our brains through food, and certain types of calories have specific effects on our brain chemicals that we actually become addicted to. These addictions form deeper nerve pathways and perpetuate themselves until we are feeding them by necessity without control. Willpower is not enough, and most people end up either surrendering to permanent obesity or going in for gastric bypass surgery.

Emotional eating can be deeply ingrained and may take more effort to get over the habit. You can see its origins in past relationships, traumas and even your upbringing. Many people fall back into "old habits" when they go back home to visit, or Mom comes over for Christmas. Others find themselves losing control when they feel familiar emotions reminding them of a past event.

Whatever the reason, these pathways can be atrophied just like any other. It might just take a little more time. Following the techniques in section one and building the skills to rewire your brain will ensure permanent success.

EFT is another good option for a shortcut on specific triggers and addictions, so when nothing else works, be sure to reference chapter eight, "Cracking your cravings code with EFT" for this highly effective technique. EFT can be your "plan B" so you always have a backup plan when the main plan isn't enough!

Seven Highly Effective Ways To Crack Your Overeating Code:

1.) Never eat in front of the TV. Watching TV causes brain function to slow in a specific way that results in a metabolic decrease to below sleeping levels. Before TV was invented, sleeping was the lowest your metabolism could drop. Certain Tibetan monks could meditate their metabolism lower than sleeping levels, but now we can rival the most trained meditation guru with a simple slouch on the couch in front of the boob tube!

Imagine how much fat you could store if you could eat in your sleep. This would be even worse than getting up for a midnight snack because your metabolism is so tanked, fat storing is automatic. Now slow it down even further with some TV viewing and you can almost hear your fat cells stretching out getting ready for the instant infusion process!

Television causes the brain to slip into alpha level where effective hypnosis takes place. This state makes you more receptive to advertisements and more likely to be convinced to buy the products. Most infomercials are not just aired at night because of the cheaper airtime rates. They are aired at night because at this time you are tired and will slip into alpha level sooner.

Images of television violence stimulate the fight or flight instinct we all have, but since it would be silly to act on this instinct, we suppress it instead. This constant stimulus and suppression cycle builds up these emotions until they are let out through events like irrational fights with our family members or even road rage.

This depicted violence also makes it harder to get to sleep when you are ready to go to bed. The inner conflict you are wrestling with from seeing those images is stirring your mood, so even if you do force yourself to sleep, that sleep is much less productive and recovery is reduced.

Television is an unnatural steady stream of information. This fractures your attention and speeds up time. This makes our perception of ordinary life dull by comparison. The reality shows exaggerate this even further with the extreme drama segments spliced together and we grow more and more discontent as our own lives seem less and less exciting by comparison.

The average American watches 5 hours of TV per day. This is effectively time spent brainwashing ourselves into becoming discontent and unsatisfied with our own lives, while increasing our desires for products we don't need, making it harder to sleep, and reducing the quality of sleep.

The happiest societies in the world are often those with the least "stuff" and technology. My father recently went on a mission trip to Mexico City to build bathrooms for the people living in the city dump. Any of us would expect to see poverty and misery beyond compare among these people, and while he did see this, he also saw kids whose happiness rivaled anything he has seen anywhere in the US.

Every year more than $50 billion is spent by the food industry and drug companies on marketing messages to U.S. consumers to influence their food and medication choices. The majority (75 percent) of commercial network television time is paid for by the 100 largest corporations in North America. Some of these companies even have advertising budgets in the billions, and not surprisingly, these budgets have the power to influence TV producers to create television that suits their agendas.

If you must watch TV, view only recorded shows and fast forward through the commercials. You can also be doing something while watching like cooking your food for the next day, yoga, crunches, stretching, etc. to make that time useful and to prevent your brain from dropping into the alpha state and slowing your metabolism to a crawl.

Many parents use their TV as a baby sitter but the consequences in the long run are always worse than the time it might buy them in the short term. TV is now believed to cause ADHD, impair your child's linguistic and social development, worsen autism, make your child fat, make them more materialistic, increase aggressiveness, and even lead to poor health choices like smoking.

A similar metabolic crash happens while in front of a computer. The typing process and thinking mechanism helps to keep it higher than watching TV, but only brings it up to about the level of sleeping. You can combat this by getting up every half hour and walking around for a minute or climbing a flight of stairs.

Most adults now spend more than 5 hours a day in front of a computer. Add the average 5 hours a day in front of the TV and then 7 hours of sleep each night, and you have a metabolism that is at or below sleeping levels for more than 17 hours out of 24 hours in a day. It's no wonder we keep getting fatter and diets keep failing us!

2.) Record everything you eat in a food log. If you commit to writing down every single thing that you eat, you will naturally eat less because your conscious and subconscious mind will not want to see it on paper.

When clients come to me and report they "eat really well" but can't lose any fat, I just have them log every liquid and solid that passes their lips for one week. Many just won't do it, so I can easily tell the ones who are serious about losing weight, but the ones that do record their foods almost always lose a pound or two in that first week even if they don't "feel" like they are doing anything different.

This phenomenon happens because they are less likely to eat "unconsciously" and forget about it because their subconscious buffers things for them. People notoriously under-report their intake—not because they are lying—but because their subconscious filters some out to make their conscious mind feel better. The food log cuts this process off and forces the connection between the conscious and subconscious.

3.) Eat only with bright lights. Restaurants have known for years that you will eat and drink more in dimly lit conditions, and less in well lit rooms. It's no mistake that fancy restaurants are usually "mood lit" with low lighting, and buffets are bright with lights everywhere.

Use this physiologic response to your advantage by turning on extra lights at meal times and eating outside on sunny days. It isn't so much the heat of the summer that makes us less hungry, it's the bright sun and longer days that are more responsible for our increased discretion.

4.) Drink water first. Your thirst mechanism is often mistranslated and confused as hunger. You might not be hungry at all, but if you are even the slightest bit dehydrated, your signals might get crossed and messages sent out to the wrong brain centers. This is especially true with chronically dehydrated people as their thirst mechanism almost always malfunctions. Water will add volume to your stomach as well, and will help send proper satiety signals when you are truly full.

5.) Eat one bite of each thing on your plate in turn and cycle between them instead of finishing one food item and then moving on to the next. Flavor varieties satiate better, so taking bites in cycles will help shut hunger down earlier.

Leaving evidence of what you just ate will help you eat less as well. Leave a little bit if each different food on your plate so you can keep a visual reminder of what you have already eaten. Research has proven that if you see evidence of what you already ate, you will feel fuller sooner.

In one such study, people who went to a sports bar could eat chicken wings free of charge and to their hearts' (or stomachs') content. Servers cleared away the bones at some tables but let the bones pile up at others. No surprise: People ate less when evidence of their feast remained front and center.

In another study, overweight people were shown how much they eat in a day by presenting the food all together, spread out on a table. They were utterly shocked! Seeing the volume, and having that mental picture, made them much more conscious of their portions from that point on.

6.) Eat in courses like the Europeans do. They get their first course right away instead of waiting and getting hungry like we do in America. They then keep getting small courses every 10-20 minutes which spreads it out over lots of time.

Europeans take their time, chew and enjoy, sip wine, and talk. This allows their hunger mechanisms to kick in and tell them to stop before overeating. They are also more able to fully digest their food.

When Americans go to a restaurant, they have to wait at least 30 minutes, are then starved, get one huge serving, and stuff it down faster than their hunger mechanism can respond.

Europeans use smaller bowls and plates as well. Americans have been programmed to finish everything on our plate, yet we have the biggest plates in the world! Europeans' plates and bowls are about half the size of Americans'.

Europeans also chew each bite thoroughly because they are taking their time. The very act of chewing contributes to satiety. The activation of your jaw muscles tells your hunger center it is being taken care of. Wolfing down food too fast skips this information passage. Chewing completely also aids digestion and helps you absorb more of the high value nutrients and less of the fats by proportion. Since your satiety center takes 15-20 minutes to register properly anyway, taking this extra chewing time will keep the volume intake down as well.

7.) Eat protein and fiber first. These fill you up fast and cause you to eat less of the stuff you know you shouldn't be eating. Protein and fiber are also high metabolic foods that attack fat stores, so the more you can get in the beginning of the meal, the better off you will be.

CHAPTER SIX

CRACKING YOUR HUNGER CODE

Our hunger sensation is a tricky bugger. Most people's hunger center doesn't work right anyway because they are either misreading it, or are chronically dehydrated. Understanding how hunger works will be the most important step towards translating your own sensations and reading them for what they really are.

There are seven types of hunger. Cellular, mass, blood sugar, volume, thirst, cilia, and emotional hunger are all various contributors to the sensation.

1.) Cellular hunger is our most instinctive hunger sensation. This hunger is caused by our cells craving certain things due to a deficiency or an addiction. If your cells are low on a certain vitamin or mineral, certain hormones will send messages to your brain that tell you to eat.

In the same way, your cells will also report low levels of addictive drugs or even certain food ingredients if the cells have become addicted to them. This will launch specific cravings or just general hunger to try to fill that void. Dehydrated cells will also cause hunger messages to be sent out which are often answered with more food consumption instead of the water they are really asking for.

When you eat certain "trigger" foods, your cells can immediately respond from the hormonal changes caused by the food and create an immediate increased craving for that food. This is the main cause for the overeating snowball effect many of us deal with on "binges." We are actually medicating ourselves with food and riding the "high" it provides.

I know it might sound redundant, but proper hydration is the biggest key to preventing overeating. Water is the best weapon to win that battle so be sure to guzzle it down before you go out to eat, or whenever you might come across your triggers, and when you feel the triggers coming on!

Cellular hunger can be a very valuable tool and even help you survive. Most of the time however, it is calling for addictive ingredients, drugs or water. When you are eating enough dark greens and protein, and drinking enough water, this type of hunger will be much more reliable and will cause you to crave healthy foods.

2.) Hormonal hunger relates to the hormones and chemicals produced in your body that cause hunger. There are many different hormones and chemicals responsible for this response so I will touch on only the main players.

Cholecystokinin (CN) is a chemical that tells your brain to stop eating. It is a short-term intense message sent via the vagus nerve to the brain. Leptin is a hormone that is more of a long-term gentle message telling your brain you are full. Eating saturated fat produces lower levels of leptin than unsaturated fat, and it doesn't stimulate CN as efficiently so you don't feel as full either.

Cocaine Amphetamine Regulatory Transcript (CART) decreases hunger and increases your metabolism. Leptin signals from your fat cells not only reduce hunger, but also simulate CART. This hormone is part of the reason many people get hot and sweaty after a big meal.

Leptin comes from your fat cells and tells you they are full so you can stop eating. When your fat cells are full and maxed out for your metabolic set point, this hormone sends its signals. If you have a high fat set point, these signals are dulled. If you have a lean set point, these signals are better received and register sooner. Alcohol inhibits leptin production and stimulates the appetite. This combined with the extra liver work and fat extraction paralysis, makes for a near perfect plan to gain fat.

The hormone ghrelin comes from the digestive system and tells you to eat more. Decreased sleep will increase ghrelin so your appetite will actually increase from poor sleep habits. You will also produce more cortisol which is a hormone that increases fat storing, so getting the proper amount of sleep is vital to balancing hormone hunger. Stress will also release cortisol and will make it harder to sleep, so active stress reduction techniques like using EFT as described in chapter eight, "Cracking your cravings code with EFT" will go a long way towards your fat burning!

Chemicals are driven by neuropeptide Y (NPY) which stimulates hunger, and increases with prolonged periods of stress. Testosterone stimulates NPY as well, which is one of the reasons men tend to have a bigger appetite than women. High intensity exercise is the best way to control NPY, CART, cortisol, and ghrelin, so make sure you are self regulating yourself internally with regular doses of intense workouts!

3.) Blood sugar levels play a very important role in your hunger. When sugar levels are low, your insulin levels will typically follow. In extreme low situations, you may even feel weak and sometimes shaky. Stomach growling can begin, your core body temperature may drop, and almost any food looks good to you.

This type of hunger can quickly be satisfied with a piece of fruit or sport drink. Most people go overboard however, and overeat or binge to make the sensation go away, because this is one of the most uncomfortable hunger sensations when it is happening. Mood swings are also common and can make rational thoughts about how much to eat go out the window.

Overeating in this case causes a rebound effect and puts you into a hyperglycemic event, causing fatigue and a heightened fat storing ability, so understanding this type of hunger and taking your feeding slow with the right kinds of foods is paramount. Try to avoid sugars and starches and stick with the lower glycemic foods to prevent the rebound effect.

This rebound is also hard on your pancreas and can even cause diabetes mellitus over time if rebounds are repeated often. The pancreas simply wears out from the extremes and stops working optimally or sometimes shuts down altogether. This damage is usually irreversible, so take care with proper habits and understanding.

Diabetes mellitus refers to a group of disorders characterized by high blood sugar and problems with blood sugar regulation. We all have blood sugar and need it for energy and many other functions ranging from thought processing to physical energy. Our blood sugar levels must be in balance for our related internal functions to work properly. Too much blood sugar can be as harmful as too little, so the body's ability to control it is vital.

The pancreas is the organ responsible for keeping blood sugar from getting too high. It does this by releasing a hormone called insulin to keep the levels down within normal operating ranges. Insulin signals the cells to take up sugar in the bloodstream and use it for internal processes and energy or store it for use later. As the cells respond to insulin and take in glucose, the levels fall and the pancreas stops releasing the hormone.

The most common type of diabetes is type 2. This disease starts gradually as people consume high levels of sugar and excess food they can't use. The result is fat gain and a pancreas that is overworked. The cells also get sick of trying to store all this extra sugar, and soon a condition known as insulin resistance sets in.

This condition is basically caused by the cells getting tired of the pancreas nagging them to store, store, store above what they are able. They start to "tune out" the pancreas much like a nagging spouse. This stage is known as "prediabetes" and is characterized by high blood sugar levels, but not high enough to qualify as diabetes. Prediabetes is often reversed with increased exercise, nutrition modification, and weight loss.

If prediabetes is not reversed, the pancreas begins to decline and reduces the amount of insulin it is releasing. The cells aren't listening anymore anyway, so it stops talking as much. It is also worn out from overworking, so reducing its workload is the natural next step. By now, the cells are used to tuning out the pancreas so their reduced sugar uptake continues. Combining that with lower insulin release from the pancreas causes diabetes to set in. Now insulin drugs or extreme nutrition habit changes are necessary.

4.) Mass related hunger has to do with the weight of the food. Your stomach senses food weight and the heavier the food, the sooner that hunger component will send its signals. This is why water and protein are so important. Water is of course, one of the heaviest materials you can put in your stomach. Protein is also heavy, and lean meats are even heavier than water.

If you want to find out for yourself the density of a certain food, just stick it in a bowl of water. If it sinks, it will be a great mass signaler. If it floats easily, it won't contribute as much to this particular signaling process.

The volume of food in your stomach will send signals to stop eating. This response is delayed however, and takes 15-30 minutes to register, so fast eating or "gorging" will skip it and rob you of this useful cue.

When we eat too fast and get too full, we feel "stretched" and very uncomfortable. Stomach stretching is actually happening here, and if repeated, will quite literally make your stomach bigger. The average empty stomach has a volume of about a liter, but can be expanded to four liters if we force it.

The stomach is very elastic, and chronic overeaters can stretch their stomachs out over time to hold as much as eight liters. The limits can be pushed even farther than this however, as demonstrated by world champion eating competitors like Kobayashi, who can eat 50 hot dogs (including buns and water) in 12 minutes!

The good news is that over time, the stomach will shrink back down with proper habits and consistency. The best way to keep your food volume in check is to take your time when you are eating. Your volume sensing center is one of your best cues to stop eating, but you have to give it time to work.

Rate your hunger on a scale of 1-10 and then only eat when you are at a 7 or higher, and stop when you get down to a 3 or 4. You might still feel hungry at a 4, but even if you stop there, you will be at a 2 or lower in another 10 minutes or less, and in 30 minutes you will be satisfied and very happy you stopped when you did! This delayed response can be anticipated, and if used to your advantage, can go a long way toward overeating prevention.

5.) Thirst response is the most often misread hunger cue. Most American are chronically dehydrated anyway, and this causes the thirst mechanism to send the wrong signals. People feel hungry when they should be feeling thirsty, because their signals are getting crossed. As you develop proper hydration habits, this mixed messaging will stop.

In the short term, you can fight this hunger miscue by drinking water 20 minutes before eating. Then reassess, and if your hunger level hasn't changed, it might very well be for another reason.

6.) Cilia hunger is an anatomically powered sensation that relates to the volume of food in your stomach. There are certain mechanisms at the top of your stomach which look like fingers sticking down that sense food when the stomach is full enough for the food to touch them. At this point, signals are sent to your brain that tell you to stop eating.

This hunger satiating response is another delayed mechanism that takes 10-20 minutes to register, so slow eating will help this work correctly as well. Some people can desensitize this response with repeated "squashing" of the cilia from overfilling the stomach. The messages also become less effective if they are sent too often with repeated overeating.

Frequent overeating stretches the stomach causing the capacity to increase, which requires more food to reach the cilia. When food volume is reduced over time, the stomach shrinks back down and the cilia response is increased. You can see how small, frequent meals help your fat loss in more ways than one!

7.) Emotional hunger is usually the most powerful sensation. We frequently medicate our brains in an attempt to alleviate stress, depression, and other emotional issues and feelings. This can be a temporary quick fix but always ends in a rebound of a worsened condition. Then the downward spiral begins until the food is part of the addiction library we store in our tissues and brain.

Some people eat when they are happy, others when they are bored, and many eat when they feel depressed, nervous, or some other common emotion. Certain hormones are released during emotional times, and these reactions can cause increased appetite and cravings that fool your body into craving certain foods when it doesn't need them at all.

Positive thoughts will help bring your hormones back in check, so simply switching your thought processes can be a quick fix to this issue. Exercise can also normalize hormones and cause chemicals to be released that actually reverse the emotional cravings. Even a short walk can reduce hunger by 20-50 percent, so any activity can help you out. High intensity exercise is especially effective in suppressing the appetite. You can notice this suppression for up to four hours, so get that workout in whenever you feel the spiral starting.

EFT can help with emotions as well as cravings, so read chapter eight, "Cracking your cravings code with EFT" thoroughly, and make sure that skill is honed as quickly as possible. Every little trick you use can add up to a big benefit in the end, so learn all the methods in this book to build up your arsenal for a permanent new you!

I really can't emphasize enough the power of EFT for curbing cravings and emotional eating. This technique can easily be your most powerful solution to permanently lose the fat you have struggled with. EFT can nip emotional eating in the bud, and cure overeating issues for life.

Cinnamon has been found to enhance the satiety center in your brain. Cooking or baking with this ingredient can actually help you reduce your portion sizes without adding any calories to the food.

Red peppers and capsaicin actually stun the hunger messages to your brain. You have probably noticed your hunger fly out the window when you eat something too hot. You go from "yum-yum" to "I'm done" in 5 seconds flat! You don't have to hurt yourself though, to shut down the hunger mechanism. Just a little spice will still work in toning down the hunger levels.

Extreme stress often turns off the hunger center in your brain as your fight or flight reflex is activated. High Intensity Training can cause this reaction as well. Even 3 minutes of intense physical output can be enough to suppress the appetite for an hour or more, which is plenty of time to eat a meal slowly, with small portions. By the time you are done eating, your fight or flight response has worn off, but because your satiety centers have now taken over from the food you ate, you aren't hungry any more, and you have just eaten much less than you would have otherwise.

Poor weather, incessant rain, and higher latitudes can cause "Seasonal Affective Disorder" (SAD) in perfectly healthy people. This is caused by too little sunlight, and the side effects of it range from depression to vitamin

D deficiency. One way to fight SAD is with a standard daily multivitamin that emphasizes Vitamin D.

Another way to fight SAD is through light therapy with full spectrum light doses of at least 10 minutes a day. Many stores and online sources have these lamps, so if you think you are a sufferer of SAD, look into this because SAD makes everything more difficult—not just a fat loss program.

Victims of SAD can have worse cravings than others because certain high-carb/high fat foods cause the release of brain chemicals that make us emotionally feel better. This feeling is of course temporary, and is usually followed by a dip lower than the original state. Finding a solution to SAD is a must. Get your Vitamin D checked by your doctor (Naturopath is best), and make sure SAD isn't sabotaging your progress!

The best technique I have found is to always plan ahead and have something prepared to eat nearby for when I get hungry. That way I am never caught hungry with nothing good to eat. It is those times when people get into trouble and just grab something quick to hold them over until they can "get enough time to make something good."

I usually do my meal prep at night before I go to bed. I make too much so it lasts me at least two days, so I'm not cooking every day. The other day I did forget to do this meal prep and remembered that I didn't have anything made for tomorrow. I was almost asleep, so instead of getting up, I set my alarm clock early and did it in the morning.

Remember that true fitness and lean bodies take commitment! If it were easy, we would all be fit and it wouldn't be anything special. Everyone would look great and no one would be a head-turner. The techniques and tips in this book just show you the easiest and fastest way to carry out this commitment.

SEVEN WAYS YOUR BODY SAYS YOU ARE HUNGRY WHEN YOU ARE NOT

Time of Day
Through routine, we condition our bodies to expect breakfast, lunch and dinner at the same time each day. Our brain clock makes a dinner bell go off whether we are truly physically hungry or not.

Sight
Research using MRI technology shows that brain patterns of people viewing photos of foods they like and foods they don't like are very different. The

body anticipates when food is about to enter the system, and that's why your mouth starts watering when you see that ad on TV.

Have you ever been crowded or pushed in line at a buffet? I sure have. It is amazing what a hurry people get in when they see a certain food. It's almost like there is a fire and they are making for the exit! These people are classic food addicts who are so taken by the sight of food, they don't even see those around them.

Variety

Even after eating a large meal and feeling full, we often "make room" for dessert, because our desire for sweets hasn't been satisfied. If you have a "salt tooth" instead, you may find yourself eating more of something salty to cap off the meal. You aren't hungry anymore, but your tongue has been programmed by you to get all its cravings filled before you stop eating.

Smell

Scent is one of the key ways we cue our bodies that food is near. Once the trigger goes off, it can induce the insulin secretion that makes us think we're hungry. Smell and sight together can really start the stampede at the buffet!

Alcohol

Alcohol will increase your appetite and it has also been shown to impair judgment, causing you to eat more. Inhibitions fall away and we tend to say, "what the heck" and have one or two more.

Temperature

The colder the temperature, the more people tend to eat, which is why restaurants often keep thermostats low. Your metabolism drops when it's time to eat because you are low on food. This often makes people cold. Eating then warms you back up, so heat is considered another satiety signal. Buffets and all-you-can-eat restaurants tend to keep their thermostat high so you eat less.

Refined Carbs

After a meal heavy in refined carbohydrates (like white pasta) the body may crave food again within only a few hours and make you eat more often. These foods cause blood sugar to drop, and this causes the blood sugar hunger to kick in that was mentioned earlier.

CHAPTER SEVEN

CRACKING YOUR SUGAR CODE

The average American consumes twenty three pounds of sugar each week. This is not surprising considering that highly refined sugars in the forms of sucrose (table sugar), dextrose (corn sugar), and high-fructose corn syrup (HFCS) are present in most processed foods.

A 20 ounce bottle of cola for instance, has a whopping 15 spoonfuls of sugar! Most soda companies don't even use straight sugar anymore. They now use HFCS which the body can't discern from refined sugar and is even *more* processed!

Twenty years ago the average person in the US ate only 8 ounces of sugar per week. In the late 1800's the average consumption was just 5 ounces per week! Cardiovascular disease and cancers were virtually unknown in the early 1900's and as you will see, there is a strong sugar connection.

One of sugar's major drawbacks which we have already discussed is that it rapidly raises your insulin level. This inhibits the release of growth hormones, which in turn depresses the immune system. Rapid insulin changes cause excess stress on the body and its organs which take away from energy normally delegated to your immune system.

We have known since the 1970's that vitamin C aids the immune system, thanks to a researcher named Linus Pauling, who found this nutrient was needed by white blood cells to destroy viruses and bacteria. White blood cells require a concentration 50 times higher inside the cell than outside, so they have to accumulate vitamin C and build it up over time.

Sugar and vitamin C have similar chemical structures, so they compete against one another to enter the cells. They also share the same mechanism that mediates the entry into the cells. If there is more sugar around, there is going to be less vitamin C allowed into the cell. It doesn't take much either, so when you eat sugar, your immune system is automatically compromised.

Since sugar is consumed in higher volumes (grams) than vitamin C (milligrams), sugar wins the battle and pushes the vitamin C out of the cell. This is why it is so sad to see "HI C" fruit punch and vitamin C "fortified" candy: the sugar present nullifies the absorption of the vitamin, so it's really just a con targeted at moms thinking they are doing their kids a favor.

Since sugar is so good at triggering insulin release, it is a great fat storage aid as well. Insulin promotes the storage of fat, so that when you eat sweets high in sugar, you're putting your body in a fat storing mode, causing rapid fat gain and elevated triglyceride levels, both of which have been linked to cardiovascular disease.

The health dangers caused by ingesting sugar on a habitual basis are undeniable. Simple sugars have been observed to cause mood swings, accelerate mental illness, cultivate gallstones, aggravate asthma, intensify nervous disorders, exacerbate heart disease, cause diabetes, increase hypertension, and worsen arthritis, to name just a few.

Because refined sugar is completely void of nutrients, it must drain and use what is already present in the body to be metabolized into the system. As nutrients are depleted, metabolization of cholesterol and fatty acid is hampered, contributing to higher triglycerides and cholesterol, which in turn promotes obesity and higher fatty acid storage around the organs and under the skin.

Sugar is the ultimate "empty calorie" substance, being one of the few ingestibles that offer absolutely zero benefits to your health and fitness. Sure it tastes good, but as a nutrient, it offers only detriments. Because it is deficient in vitamins, minerals and fiber, and has such a deteriorating effect on the endocrine system, major health organizations (American Dietetic Association and American Diabetic Association) agree that its consumption in America is one of the three top causes of degenerative disease.

Besides the health complications listed above, sugar has been proven to have a direct and causative correlation on the following conditions:

- **Inflammation**. Any current injuries, tendonitis, joint, or muscle pain is increased by consuming sugar. It even prevents healing in some cases because it fights against the body's natural ability to reduce the inflammation cycle.
- **Wrinkles and grey hair** due to free radical production caused by processing sugar.
- **Eczema and acne** from sugar induced hormone imbalances.

- **Kidney damage**: Besides the extra unnecessary load on the kidneys to rid the body of excess sugar, the adrenal glands work closely with the kidneys, so the extra strain on them causes even more problems for the kidneys.
- **Tooth decay**: Everyone knows sugar decays the teeth and here's the proof: the only animal besides humans who *always* has tooth decay problems is the honey bear!
- **Acid stomach symptoms and ulcers.** Sugar has a direct and immediate causative effect on these symptoms, but also has a long-term effect on acid reflux as it encourages internal fat gain. This fat changes the routing of your digestive tubes that drastically exacerbates the problem.
- **Migraines and other headaches** are often caused by brain chemical imbalances and sugar buildup.
- **Osteoporosis** can be caused from reduced mineral absorption.
- **Decreased mental clarity and memory** function often result due to an increase in alpha, delta, and theta brain waves.
- **Increased risk of blood clots and strokes.**
- **Increased bacterial fermentation** in the colon.
- *CANCER*: Otto Warburg, Ph.D., the 1931 Nobel laureate in medicine discovered that *cancer cells run on sugar*. Starving the cancer cells of their preferred fuel source slows their growth, and can even help kill them off. Reducing sugar also allows the immune system to operate optimally. It is no coincidence that in every successful alternative cancer treatment center in the world, sugar is completely eliminated from the diet as the very first step.

The only time I have been sick (even with a minor head cold) *in the last four years* was during a holiday season when I let myself eat whatever I wanted. I did it as an experiment and expected to gain fat, but what I didn't count on was becoming ill. I also noticed my mental clarity, memory and even speech patterns were affected drastically. This reminded me just how toxic sugar really is.

No one is telling you to cut sugar out of your diet immediately. If you do that you will just crave it more. It is a physically addictive substance, so weaning yourself is not easy. The best thing to do is just reduce the amount slowly over time and limit your consumption progressively each day.

Try to avoid artificial sweeteners too (including Splenda/Sucralose). These are just as bad for your health as sugar and in some cases, even worse. In fact, some studies show that consuming products that contain artificial sweeteners may actually encourage you to eat more servings than you would if the food or drinks were sweetened with real sugar.

Sugar substitutes interfere with the body's natural ability to perceive intake volumes based on a food's sweetness. When this ability is skewed, you will be more likely to overeat than if you just had real sugar!

One guaranteed healthy sweetener alternative is Stevia. This can be found at any whole food or supplement store and is made from the Stevia plant with no refining involved. Since it requires such a small amount (100 times less than sugar), it contributes no calories and has no effect on insulin levels.

If you want to accelerate your fitness, increase your immune system, improve your health, and prevent disease, start cutting down your sugar. Doing it in steps will make success and adherence much more likely. Make it a lifestyle decision and you will reap the benefits forever!

CHAPTER EIGHT

CRACKING YOUR CRAVING CODE WITH EFT

This chapter describes a handy little technique to permanently break certain addictions you struggle with. These addictions can range from food, to alcohol, to emotional eating, and more. It is called EFT (Emotional Freedom Technique) and was popularized by Gary Craig (*www.emofree. com*). This technique follows along the same lines as acupressure and even acupuncture in some ways, but involves only tapping with your fingers on certain points instead of pinching or poking.

EFT is based on a new discovery that has provided thousands with relief from pain, diseases and emotional issues. Simply stated, it is an emotional version of acupuncture except needles aren't necessary. Instead, you stimulate well established energy meridian points on your body by tapping on them with your fingertips. The process is easy to memorize and can be done anywhere.

Since it acts on the nerve pathways in your brain, you don't have to believe it will work for it to be effective. It works just as well on skeptics as it does on converts. There are no negative side effects either, so if it works for you, there will be only benefits.

Every thought, emotion, craving, memory and addiction is simply a specific nerve pathway in your brain. The more often you travel that pathway, the deeper it gets. I touched on this earlier in the book by explaining how food addictions get worse during a diet even though that food has been avoided the whole time.

It is important to be "in the craving" for this to be the most effective. The rest of this book talks about switching over nerve pathways and thinking about what you should be eating every time you think about your "bad" food craving, but for this technique you should actually go with your craving so you can disrupt the nerve pathway electrically.

You will interrupt that craving nerve pathway as it is being traveled and will be permanent. It is kind of like a short circuit in the brain for that specific impulse and the EFT "burns it out." It doesn't work on everyone, but for the vast majority, it is quite effective. As of the printing of this book, I have so far experienced a 100% success rate with the many people I have taught it to.

Another nice thing about EFT is that it usually only takes 1-3 minutes to perform. I even use it at stop lights with success. It also is a skill that gets better with use, so frequent practice only increases its effectiveness.

I know you are probably eager to get started learning this easy method, so I'll save more explanations for later and get right to the training. I will only explain the "shortcut" to you here, but if you want more extensive training or find it ineffective, you can visit the EFT website for more tips and tricks that might work better.

The tapping points are listed below, so familiarize yourself with them first. Some points may be more effective for you than others and you will learn this with practice and time. Each tapping point should be tapped with two fingers 7-10 times for about 5 seconds.

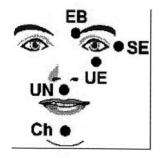 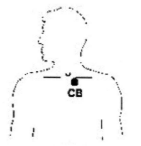 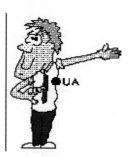

As you are feeling the craving, say the phrase, "this _____ craving" (i.e. "this chocolate craving") as you lightly tap each point. It doesn't matter which side of your face or body you tap, or even if you mix it up. It also doesn't matter in which order you tap the points. After you tap through all 7 points, reflect for a moment on your craving and see if it is reduced. Rate it on a scale of 1-10 before you start tapping and rate it again after each tapping cycle.

Sometimes it will reduce to a one or zero on the first attempt and other times it will only go down a point or two. If it reduces only slightly, repeat the cycle and use the phrase, "this remaining _____ craving."

If you find no progress at all, you might be "psychologically reversed" and need to do what is called the "setup." If you are psychologically reversed, your subconscious mind is not ready yet to give this thing up even though your conscious mind thinks you are. The setup will align your subconscious with your conscious mind and help prepare your brain to receive the information and nerve disruption more effectively.

The setup involves finding a sore spot on your upper chest first. Poke around for a while and see if you can find a spot that is sorer than other areas. This is a lymph congestion area and you will keep your fingers there while you massage it lightly to break it up. If you can't find it on one side, try the other. Either side will work fine.

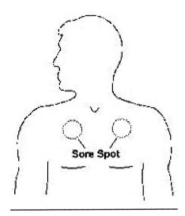

As you lightly massage this area in a circular pattern, say the phrase, "Even though I have this _____ craving, I deeply and completely accept myself." I know this sounds corny, and it is, but the more you try to mean it, the better it will work to get your brain ready to receive the signal disruption. You are effectively patting your subconscious on its little head and telling it to relax and listen up.

After performing the setup, cycle through the tapping points and craving phrase again. If you now have movement downward on the rating scale, you are no longer psychologically reversed, and will continue to see reduction in the craving intensity with each successive attempt.

You will sometimes get to a zero on your craving scale with one or two tapping cycles. Sometimes there are other aspects as well preventing full reduction to a zero. This is OK because even getting to a one or two is usually far enough to cross it off your craving list.

The most trouble I had with anyone took him from a 9 down to a 5 on his craving scale, but that was enough of a reduction for him to resist it next time with his own willpower. He later reduced it even further through using the other principles in this book which caused that particular pathway to just wither away from disuse over time.

I know it sounds complicated, but the bottom line is every craving that you have is a nerve impulse or pathway in your brain. These impulses can be very deep if they have been traveled for a long time. No matter how deep it is however, any pathway can be broken. Between EFT and the regular practice of the brain wiring techniques in this book, success will be 100% for your case as well.

Most cravings are rooted in an emotion, not the certain food. The food you crave in response to an emotion, does specifically cause release of certain hormones to help you with that mood, but the effects are always short term, cyclic, and very chemically addictive.

The habit that forms can be even worse, and turns into a whole new nerve pathway that forms as a result of the original emotional "trigger." We all succumb to emotional eating. Even I find myself being fooled into thinking I'm hungry (when I'm really not), if my emotions are ripe enough from certain situations.

EFT saves me from emotional eating 3-5 times a week on average. Because EFT is a skill and its effectiveness is improved with practice, I'm very good at it, so it only takes me 20-40 seconds to cure myself of emotional eating cravings.

This is my single most effective tool for avoiding unnecessary eating and could easily be the whole answer to your emotional eating problem as well. Just simply tap the emotion you are feeling that makes you feel hungry. Mine is usually stress, so I just say, "This stress" while I am tapping.

I also know that anger releases chemicals and hormones in me that break me down, so I tap for that as well. Anger is the opposite of happiness and contentment, so I try to nip anger in the bud as soon as I feel it coming on.

At any given moment, you are either spiraling up along a positive path of improvement and optimism, or spiraling down towards negativity and ill health. There is no in between. EFT can stop the negative emotions and downward spiral, so you can regain control and spiral upward without the need for extraordinary amounts of willpower!

CHAPTER NINE

CRACKING THE SUPPLEMENT CODE

Supplements are so confusing because most of the information we get is from supplement companies telling us we need their product. They even cite "research" studies to prove that they are the best, but most of those are done by the companies themselves or a biased source that claims to be "independent."

Here is the bottom line: you don't need supplements. You can get all your nutrient needs through food. Just look at the early fitness and bodybuilders as an example. They looked fantastic and felt even better, but did not have access to supplements or steroids because they didn't exist yet! Physique superstars like Steve Reeves and Rachel McLish did it with good old fashioned exercise and real food.

Supplements only help if you don't follow proper nutritional guidelines. If you feel better from taking a supplement, it's probably because you are suffering from deficiencies in your diet. The supplement will add in nutrients you aren't supplying your self with naturally from food, and you feel the improvement. Most Americans actually do benefit from supplements, but that just shows how poor the typical diet is.

If you find a magic supplement, metabolic enhancer, or diet pill that works like a charm, it's probably due to the placebo effect. You believe it will work and so it does. Because of this belief, you make conscious and unconscious decisions throughout the day that make the pill work. Just the act of taking the pill reminds you of your new commitment to lose fat, so you eat better without knowing you are even doing it.

The product itself isn't doing squat, but the physical act of putting the pill in your mouth reminds you that you want to get leaner that day. The products that require you to take the pill 3 times a day or with a meal are even more effective because you are thinking about it more often and eating better and less food at your meals. The flip side of that however, is that you are also reminding yourself that you can't do it on your own, and reinforcing the notion of failure. This guarantees the rebound weight to come back on when you are done with the pill treatments.

Even if a product accurately claims no side effects, the rebound effect due to the psychological reinforcement of failure and product dependency can be the most severe side effect of them all. It can also be more permanent because you are changing your brain wiring in the wrong direction!

Most supplement companies claim to be "magic bullets" with the answer to all your weight loss dreams. They market them in a way that convinces you of their effectiveness so the placebo effect makes them work. Your belief in a metabolism increase can actually cause one. That is how powerful your brain is! When you stop taking the product however, your belief stops as well and the changes back to baseline come with it.

Many diet pill manufacturers also ship their product with their own diet program as an added "bonus." This program is probably better than your own nutrition habits, so you will most likely get results by following it, but then you attribute all the fat loss to their pill instead of their program.

The supplement manufacturer counts on this and hopes you will follow their lifestyle changes along with taking their product, because they know darn well their product doesn't work worth squat. As long as you believe it is their pill that is giving you the results, you will keep ordering it from them.

The down side is that you never developed a permanent brain change because you were depending on the supplement and were giving it all the credit. By doing this, you never changed any nerve pathways in your brain, and the result is a rebound back to where you started, or worse.

Save your money and just do the mental steps in the beginning chapter of this book! I haven't found a fat burner that works or a supplement (besides protein powder) that produces any real results yet. If there was a product that gave true results, the FDA would ban it or have control over it and you would only be able to get it through prescription. If it is available over the counter, it probably is just a waste of money and will cause side effects that will outweigh any benefit (physiological or not).

I must confess that I do use supplements, but not for the reasons you might expect. Most of the supplements I take are experimental. I have tried every legal and healthy supplement out there to test the manufacturer's claims. If I am to endorse a product or deny its effectiveness, I need to experience it personally, so I try it out first.

To date, I have not experienced success with any supplement of any kind besides regular protein powders. I will address the top supplements here and discuss their effectiveness to save you some time and money.

Protein powders: I use a natural protein powder sweetened with Stevia, because I have no appetite in the morning for breakfast, and I know I need to get something in me to shut off the muscle burning in the morning and continue the fat burning zone that starts each day. I also will occasionally make another protein shake after a workout if I am not hungry enough for food.

The two most important times of the day for protein are in the morning and after a workout. When you wake up, you are automatically in a tissue burning state due to the fact that you have been fasting all night. You metabolism has tanked, and you are feeding off of your muscle and fat.

You can shut down the muscle burning mode but continue the fat burn by taking in protein without carbs. You will easily absorb the protein in the absence of carbs because you are highly anabolic in the morning as your body is looking for any nutrients it can find.

Eating only protein for breakfast like a whey shake, eggs, meat, etc., will stop the muscle burning mode but encourage the fat burning mode to continue on. Your morning metabolism dip will also be reversed, since protein is such a high metabolic food. The combination of the continuation of your fat burning mode along with the increased metabolism will actually help elevate the amount of fat you burn during this morning window.

Another time protein is easily absorbed and more fat will be burned off, is right after a high intensity workout. Like the morning time, your body is looking for any nutrients after vigorous exercise, so giving it protein is ideal. The research says to consume it within 5 minutes of exercise so drinking it during, right before, or immediately after exercise will fill this window just fine. Try it all three ways and see which agrees with you the best.

There is recent compelling evidence that suggests a 20 gram shot of whey protein right before going to sleep will increase release of natural growth hormone (HGH) during the night. This is significant because HGH levels decline with age and this decline is associated with many aging effects. Elevating HGH naturally can reverse or slow the signs of aging.

HGH is a buzzword now days because many people are taking synthetic forms to feel young again. Doctors claim it is safe, but that's what they said about steroids back in the 70's and we all know how that turned out. If you could find a way to release it naturally, wouldn't that be the preferred choice? It wouldn't hurt to try this 20 gram shot experiment, and might even help.

Whey protein is the most biologically active protein and easiest for the body to absorb. It is also the fastest absorbing protein and is one of the world's oldest 'health foods'. Hippocrates, known as the 'Father of Medicine', recommended the health-boosting benefits of whey in 420 B.C. In Europe during the middle ages, whey was regarded as a health tonic. Modern scientists are now discovering an amazing array of additional healthful benefits from whey.

The first protein source you were designed to eat as a newborn was mother's milk. It is no coincidence that the single most important nutritional protein in the first meal of your life was whey protein. In fact, mothers' milk is 70% whey.

Vitamins: With a balanced diet, you won't need them. If you must take a vitamin, just take a multivitamin. Formulas for men and women are more specific, and a general multivitamin tab is just fine. If you are eating healthy and balanced meals however, you won't need it and the extra will just be excreted, so you will only be wasting your money. People who travel or eat out often because of their job may find it harder to have optimal nutrition habits, so they may need a multivitamin as an insurance policy to get their nutrient requirements.

Taking individual vitamins or mega dose packs of certain vitamins can actually work against you. Correct combinations of certain vitamins are crucial and getting too much of one can block absorption of another. Vitamin D for example, may be needed for those who live in higher latitudes and have a hard time manufacturing their own from sunlight. For those people a supplement might be necessary, but certain types of vitamin D are better than others, and amounts must be balanced with calcium and other micronutrients for proper absorption. Be sure to ask your naturopath for tips on your physiology and how to optimize your intake of this and other vitamins.

Mega dosing certain vitamins and minerals can be dangerous as well. Fat soluble vitamins can build up in your system and cause toxicity which can lead to some serious health problems. The USRDA (minimum recommended daily allowances for vitamins and minerals) on the other hand, is typically too low for optimal health. The USRDA is merely the minimum requirement for an average person to prevent disease. Meeting these minimum levels will probably keep you from getting scurvy, beriberi, or some nasty deficiency symptom, but will not meet your requirements to thrive.

I'm not going to go into the minimal and maximal requirements for individuals because they are very specific to each person's physiology and conditions. They also vary greatly between men and women and change with height, weight, age, climate, pregnancy, certain diseases, and activity levels, to name just a few of the many variables.

You can ensure that you are getting the right amounts, with the correct balance for optimal absorption, through eating real food from organic sources. The most nutrient dense foods on the planet are dark green vegetables like broccoli, spinach, kale, and collard greens, to name just a few. Make sure you are eating plenty dark vegetables every day and you will be absorbing all the vitamins you need in the right ratios and correct amounts.

Protein bars: I have yet to find a healthy bar with the right balance of protein, carbs and fat. If I do find an organic real food bar, the carbs are too high and the protein is too low to be classified as a protein bar. The others are full of sugar, artificial sweeteners, or high fructose corn syrup.

Protein bars are fine in small amounts but not as a staple. The body won't recognize them as real food so it won't absorb them as completely. Your body might even keep you in starvation mode and at a lower metabolism in spite of the bar, as it waits for real food.

Eating the majority of calories in supplements and bars can make you gain weight and become malnourished even if the macronutrient ratio is exactly the same as the same calorie volume in real food.

If you must eat a protein bar now and then, only do so in emergency situations when you don't have a better option. Make sure it is a whole food bar, and if you can, find one with protein as the biggest number on the nutrition label.

If you find yourself reaching for a protein bar, reach for natural beef jerky or a chunk of meat you have prepared instead. I will often go for some organic cottage cheese, string cheese, or roll some natural lunch meat and organic cheese slice together as a better option as well.

Creatine: This product was designed to help people workout harder so they can get more out of their exercise. Studies show conflicting results, but among people with low pain tolerances, creatine might actually help them squeeze out an extra rep or two. The risks associated with creatine have been much more well documented than the benefits, however. This product is certainly not worth trying, no matter how much "safer" a particular manufacturer claims their form is than the competition.

Thermogenics: This class of supplement claims to speed up your metabolism and burn off more fat. Some also claim to be an appetite suppressant. Their ingredients vary greatly but many contain caffeine, certain herbs, and/or Ephedra (ephedrine). These products have come on and off the market because of potential dangers and negative side effects.

The bottom line is that it's just not worth the risk. People have actually died from such products. I even have a friend who lost her dog to a horrible painful death because he got into her product. Anything that can violently kill a dog (much like the way rat poison would) probably isn't too good for people either.

I've tried some but skipped over most of them due to the potential dangers. I hear reports on all of them however, from those who have tried them, and the overwhelming consensus is that they do certainly make people feel jittery, nervous and anxious, but do not provide the results promised in the marketing materials.

Bitter orange extract has been marketed as a fat loss supplement and appetite suppressant but with no real studies to confirm its effectiveness. Because it contains synephrine, a drug similar to ephedrine, it can have negative side effects ranging from anxiety to stroke or heart problems. I have not tried this due to the potential risk.

Ginger is believed by some to have thermogenic effects but there is no compelling evidence to support the claims. Ginger has other health benefits as well, so it might be a good idea to consume it as long as you aren't allergic and it won't conflict with any medications you might be taking. Ask your naturopath for their opinion of this and any other supplement you may be considering, no mater how safe you might think it might be.

Capsicum is a hot pepper that has been shown to provide temporary metabolic elevation. It's pretty hot though, so cooking with it might not be worth it. Finding it in capsule form might be a more reasonable way to go. The effects are fairly temporary however, so for the 30 minutes or so of metabolic elevation it provides, it might not be worth the cost. I have tried it and have not experienced additional fat loss benefits.

Brown seaweed has shown some possible promise in the preliminary scientific research so far. It is thought to be a natural metabolism booster and fat burner with no negative side effects. In fact, it has some additional health benefits as well. When shopping for this product, it is important to do your homework on how it is produced and what quality control system is used to preserve the integrity and potency. If you just go for the cheap stuff, you probably won't be buying the most effective form. I have taken this product with no metabolism or fat loss benefits.

Green tea has also been found to raise the metabolism and burn off fat. Some think it has more to do with the natural caffeine found in it, but others think it is due to the plant itself. It has some antioxidant qualities and brain health benefits as well, so I do take it for those reasons, but I have not found it to have any effects on fat loss.

Appetite suppressants: This one has been around longer than most weight loss supplements. They vary greatly in type and ingredients. Some actually work pretty well but when you go off of them, you go back to normal, so long term benefits can't be expected. Most come with negative side effects, so the risk makes it not worth the trouble and expense.

Hoodia may be the exception to this rule. This plant extract does seem to naturally take away your desire to eat, without any known side effects. It is thought to mimic the effects of glucose on your brain, making you feel full.

The Bushmen of the Kalahari Desert have been eating the hoodia plant for centuries. They eat natural foods of course, so weight control wasn't the purpose of eating hoodia, but when food was scarce, they would use it to reduce their hunger pains.

It was first researched in the 1960s as part of a study about indigenous foods. Researchers noticed the animal test subjects ate less when given hoodia, which resulted in weight loss. It wasn't until the 90's when the active ingredient was identified that acted as the appetite suppressant.

Now it is available from different manufacturers and in different quality gradients. Some manufacturers don't have good enough quality control, or include amounts too small to have an effect, while others provide the right amounts in proper quantities.

If you take hoodia, make sure you use it only as a temporary supplement of last resort and don't let it become a crutch! If you depend on it and ignore the brain technique exercises, it will only be a temporary fix and the weight will come back on as you come back off of it.

Hoodia might be a good idea for morbidly obese individuals who are on the verge of gastric bypass surgery. In that case, I would recommend hoodia over the surgery option as long as psychological methods are employed while taking the supplement so the brain can change in the right direction as the weight is lost. Realizing the temporary effects and using the techniques in the beginning of this book should be enough to prevent the rebound effect when hoodia is no longer needed.

The other problem with appetite suppressants is that they reduce your intake of good nutrients as well. You will probably just eat the same junk you did before, just less of it. You will also eat less of the foods that may have been good for you (like protein and greens) and now that you are eating less of those too, you are losing ground from a nutrient standpoint and are probably losing muscle as well.

The best appetite suppressant I have found is water sweetened with EmergenC and Stevia. EmergenC is a product that comes in a powder packet and has vitamins and minerals in it, but also contributes some flavor to the water. Stevia adds more sweetness, and together with the volume of water and hydration properties, satisfies mass hunger, hydration hunger, volume hunger, cellular hunger, and sweetness hunger.

Apples have been shown through research to reduce the amount eaten at a meal as well. When consumed 10-20 minutes before eating, people tend to eat less at the meal. This is due to the fiber in the apple as well as the sweetness value and nutrient contribution.

I touched on gastric bypass surgery earlier and want to revisit that topic (even though it is not a supplement) because I feel this decision is a very important one. There are several forms of gastric bypass surgery, but they all accomplish the same goal, which is to make the stomach smaller so you eat less.

The biggest problem is that nutrient absorption is drastically reduced due to the corresponding low food intake. It is hard to get the minimum required nutrients through this small stomach unless the bypass patient is willing to eat only dark greens and meat. If they are, they didn't need the surgery, because they would have been able to lose all the weight eating this way in the first place.

Most people who choose the permanent gastric procedures, end up taking vitamin and mineral supplements for the rest of their lives to get their required minimum nutrients. This takes more effort and commitment than doing the brain techniques in the beginning of this book, so the easier healthier way is obvious here.

Most bypass patients keep eating the same things as before, but must reduce the amount they eat, so they lose weight from volume decreases. Since it is more like a crash diet, they lose muscle along with the fat, so they aren't helping their metabolism out at all. In fact, they are just permanently slowing it down.

Some procedures are reversible after the weight is off, but unless the patient gets the proper mental changes accomplished, they will just rebound back up with the same nutrition habits as before. The brain has to change along with the body if the body is to stay lean after the weight loss has been accomplished.

After the reversal surgery, patients then have the extra step of gaining their muscle back without gaining fat back. Losing weight without surgery can skip this very difficult step and is always much more permanent.

There are many other risks to gastric surgery besides malnutrition, so research it carefully. My recommendation is of course, to opt out and avoid this procedure at all costs.

CHAPTER TEN

CRACKING THE DIET CODE

Perricone, Blood Type, Body Type, Pritikin, Atkins, South Beach, Maple Syrup Diet, Grapefuit Diet, Astrology Diet, Detox Diets, and low fat diets are just a few of the diets that have come out in recent years. I could go into each diet specifically, but the bottom line is that if a particular one works or you, it's probably because you are simply eating better than you used to.

You may have asked yourself why some people respond well to certain diets and others don't. Everyone's physiology is different and unique and will respond differently than someone else's. Most diets will also get you to a point and then leave you on an indefinite fat loss plateau where nothing seems to budge.

A restrictive or "crash" diet to lose weight fast is never a good idea for anyone. These diets will always cause muscle loss along with fat loss. In restrictive diets, the muscle lost can be even more than the fat lost. Since muscle is your metabolism, losing it will reduce your metabolism. This combined with the increased cravings from depriving yourself of certain foods almost always results in a fast weight rebound after the diet is over.

The rebound weight is mostly fat too, so even if you only got back to your previous weight, you are much worse off because you have less muscle than you did before the diet started and your metabolism is now weaker as well.

Fasting and most cleansing diets always burn muscle and screw up your metabolism, so avoid these drastic nutritional practices as well. Fasting can sometimes be for religious reasons, so make that your only exception. Just know that fasting or any vastly restrictive diet will burn muscle and reduce your metabolism which will always send you in the wrong direction.

Weight loss while fasting is much like weight loss when you are ill. Sickness usually results in dehydration and a reduced appetite, so muscle is at risk of being broken down for energy. Your fat storage ability is also blocked when you feel achy, so significant fat can also be lost when you are sick.

Fat that is lost rapidly is gained back fast because your body is used to having it, so crash diets cause rebounds more easily than slow fat loss. The rapid muscle loss during a crash diet however, is not gained back as rapidly because it is a high metabolic tissue that takes more time to build and rebuild.

Therefore, the weight is gained back (or more) but mostly from fat since the body is trying to guard against another food deficit. Your body thought it was in a famine—not on a diet, so it improves its fat storing ability in case another famine comes along. Since muscle is a high maintenance tissue and requires a lot of energy and calories to maintain it, your body tries to gain less of this back to make itself more efficient for the next famine as well.

Every time this cycle happens, your body gets better at losing muscle and worse at losing fat. It also gets worse at gaining muscle back, and it becomes more skilled at gaining fat back. This makes it harder to lose fat without losing muscle in subsequent attempts because your body has become so good at losing both. It forgot how to lose only fat and has to relearn that process.

Eventually it will relearn how, and will even get to the point where it can lose fat and GAIN muscle at the same time. Teaching it to do this requires some patience along with consistent healthy nutrition practices and regular strength training. This consistency is the key.

If you consistently teach your body that famines occur regularly with repeated crash diets, it will adapt to that. This cycle turns into a syndrome that spirals downward until the result is a broken metabolism that is very hard to fix.

This by itself would be bad enough, but the real destructive part of this process is what is happening to the brain. Nerve pathways are being formed that encourage the downward spiral, and your addictions and cravings are being cultivated and strengthened. These physical and mental factors combine to create a syndrome that is often permanent with little hope of escape.

Rapid fat loss can even be dangerous for some people. Obese individuals have more than a 50% chance of developing gallstones when they lose weight fast. An overworked liver caused by being overweight makes more bile, and when fat is lost rapidly, the liver doesn't empty out fast enough and makes gallstones.

Losing fat the right way is about the walk, not the sprint. It means walking the walk for life instead of a short temporary sprint across a finish line. Slow and steady also requires more time, and this allows you to adjust mentally along the way so when you reach your goals, you are changed both physically and mentally. Changing both ways is the only way to ensure success.

Fad diet programs also use clever marketing materials like case histories and radical before and after pictures that "prove" the diet's effectiveness. Many of these pictures aren't even real and some are procured from contests the diet founder creates to pump up their marketing.

I know of one exercise and diet system that has a contest every year with big prize money to the one who has the biggest physical transformation. They get about 100,000 people to enroll in the contest, but only about 2% end up finishing it and sending in their "after" pictures. That is not a great success rate by any measure, but out of the 2,000 pictures sent in at the end, there are a couple dozen that look pretty good. Those of course are the ones used on the cover of the book and marketing material, so everyone who sees it assumes that is how it will turn out for them too. What they don't see is the 99.9% who failed miserably.

The funny thing is that most of the people who failed still think the program is right for them. The marketing is so good, they still think it will work even though their own personal experience has proven otherwise. People come to me all the time raving about a certain diet and I just ask them how it has worked for them so far. That of course stumps them and helps them realize they have bought into a scam.

Even if a diet is a good one, commitment is really the biggest key to making it work effectively. Most people think they are doing a diet well, but because their current habits creep into it, they end up doing their own "modified version." Then when it doesn't work, they blame it on the diet instead of accepting that they really didn't give it a good shot.

Water is really hot at 80% boiling temperature (170 degrees). It's still hot at 99.9% of boiling (211 degrees), but it doesn't boil until it's at 100% boiling temperature (212 degrees). The same goes for your metabolism and fat loss results. If you are sticking to the plan 80% of the time, you can expect about 50% of the results you want (at best). If you are running at 99.9% commitment, you can expect pretty good results, but only 100% commitment always produces 100% results.

Some people might even crank it up to 211 degrees of commitment and start to see some good results, but only those who follow it perfectly with full commitment and 212 degrees will discover if a certain diet really works for them or not. This doesn't mean you have to be perfect every day for the rest of your life. No one is. It just means that every perfect day is a huge step toward your goals, so pat yourself on the back and affirm to yourself that you can do it when you have these days!

Some of the diets listed above are actually pretty healthy, but ask yourself if it is a diet that is designed to stick with for life, and if you are committed 212 degrees to that end. Most diets are too complicated for this however, and require too much thought and effort so they are hard to adopt and stick with permanently.

I know a diet that will work for everyone. I hesitate to even call it a diet because it really is just a lifestyle change and permanent nutritional overhaul. If you are committed to a lifelong nutritional change, you can save yourself some trouble and just start eating healthier now. It really is easier than you think.

Diets are usually thought of as temporary and are used to get weight off fast. Then when you go off the diet, you rebound back up to where you were (or worse) because your mindset hasn't changed. If you just focus on the following 7 things, you will lose all the weight you need to permanently, and you can stick with it for life.

- Have the right mental focus
- Drink enough water
- Get plenty of protein
- Go crazy for dark green vegetables
- Find organic food sources
- Get plenty of exercise
- Improve the quality of your sleep

This of course sounds simple, and it is. It's nothing really new and innovative, like most of the other things in this book, because it's basically just common sense. This is how we ate before we had sugar, and we got along just fine. We also got along just fine before ovens and baked goods came along about 3000 years ago.

I'm not saying we all have to stop eating baked goods, sugar, or skip enjoying the family holiday feasts. I'm simply saying that there are a few basic foods that can give every personality, blood type, and body type all the nutrition we need. We are just making it too complicated!

These few basic foods might sound pretty boring, but with the vast amounts of spices, cooking styles, and combinations, the options really are only as limited as we allow them to be.

Getting to the point of accomplishing these permanent lifestyle changes is different for all of us however. Some people can do them all at once and never look back but most of us need to take it in steps.

Don't be in a hurry either. Take your time. You have the rest of your life to accomplish this, so go at your own pace. If you set out from the beginning to make these changes permanent, you will be able to focus with the right attitude and form the permanent nerve changes in your brain necessary to make the new you inside as well as outside.

Slow changes are OK because fast changes can cause problems in and of themselves like strengthening addictions or even causing gallstones as mentioned earlier. Slow changes in phases are more likely to be permanent as well. Fast changes are almost always temporary with catastrophic setbacks and rebounds.

Many people try a diet for a month or so and then give up because they don't see any results. Their focus isn't permanent. It's on a quick fix weight loss that is temporary from the start. Everyone will experience plateaus in fat loss as well. This is a natural way the body loses fat and is to be expected. Understanding the body's natural resistance to weight loss-especially the initial plateau and subsequent plateaus, will help you get through these periods. If you just wait them out, you will win in the end.

Certain personality types take to some diets better than others. I have found that for checklist type people, a good initial phase is starting this way:

Before 5 pm eat whatever you want but make sure you get the following quotas:

- three servings of protein (one serving is the size of your fist)
- 80 oz. of water
- two servings of vegetables (one serving is the size of your fist)

After 5 pm eat as much as you want of only the following three items:

- White meat
- Deep dark greens (spinach, kale, collard greens, broccoli, etc.)
- Water

Try this plan three days a week and see what happens. When you are good at it, add another day. Give this or any nutrition modification at least two months because your initial plateau might fight you that long. This plan puts the focus on what you should be eating instead of what you shouldn't be eating so it trains your brain as well as your body.

On the days you are following the plan, have 100% commitment. Do not add another day unless you are perfect on the days you commit to. This will reinforce the 212 degree analogy already mentioned and will carry over to the days you do add when you are ready.

If I had a dime for every person who gave up because they cheated once, I'd have quite the stack of dimes! Cheating can also be an unconscious excuse to give up completely. Many people set themselves up for failure because they expect to, by telling their subconscious that will happen. We all usually get what we expect, so expect success and have faith that it will work!

Many people use the term "fell off the wagon" when they "cheat" with a food they know they shouldn't eat. I tend to think of it as falling off a train rather than a wagon, because if you fall off a wagon, you have to run to catch up to it if you want to get back on. This is mentally discouraging because it perpetuates the thought of having to catch up with extra effort.

If you fall off of train, it is still beside you and still moving, so if you get back on, you still get to the station at the end—you just get there later than if you had stayed on the whole time. The train station at the end is your goal and when you reach it, you have won.

Falling off the train is human. I have never met one person who didn't fall off more than once. The whole key however, is to hop back on as soon as possible! Most people will wallow in their failure and beat themselves up about falling off. Some even cheat more and say the heck with it for that day.

Cheating and then thinking "this day is blown, I'll just keep cheating and then be extra good tomorrow" is very mentally damaging. This is like falling off the train and then walking backwards. Tomorrow comes and you have all that lost progress in the back of your mind making it harder to climb back on.

This just takes more time and keeps you from making progress toward the station. The train is still going; you're just not on it. The faster you stop feeling sorry for yourself and get back on, the sooner you will get to the station.

Remember that everything you do is immediately history. If you fall off, put it behind you and get back on. Self pity, sabotage behavior, and regret only keep you off the train longer. If you can get right back on, you've only missed out on a couple of box cars and your arrival time won't really be that much later.

You might also find yourself jumping on and off the train frequently. You get back on fast, but you jump back off fast too. This of course delays your arrival accordingly, but if you keep trying, forgiving yourself, and putting it behind you each time, you will get better at riding that train. The jump offs will become less frequent and the jumps back on will get easier and quicker.

When you find yourself consistent with this plan and you are fully committed for 7 days per week, the next step is to move the cutoff time. Try moving it from 5 pm to 4 pm. When that isn't such a big deal, move it to 3 and so on as far as you are comfortable, and at your own pace.

When someone sees what I eat each day, they consider me a fanatic. It took a while to get to that point however. When I was a kid, I pretty much survived on sugar cereal for breakfast, PB&J sandwiches for lunch, a bag of Doritos (family size) after school, and Hamburger Helper for dinner. I couldn't be more opposite from that today.

Even as recently as 2006, I wasn't eating well consistently. I did fine most of the time, but was still experimenting with different foods and macronutrient combinations. I was also trying to gain fat so I could try different experiments in losing it, so everything was pretty inconsistent.

I also hadn't formed the nerve pathways I have now, so eating right wasn't as easy either. Now I know how to do it right and since I have been consistent now for some time, it's easy as well. My brain pathways make it easy to stick with my present patterns without the need for willpower, and my cells crave the nutrients they get every day through the good foods I eat.

I am now repulsed by sugar foods because of the way they make me feel. I am so detoxified, that when I do eat them, I feel horrible. My cravings have changed as well. My past uncontrollable cravings for chips and brownies have actually been replaced with cravings of the same intensity for foods like grass-fed beef and broccoli!

Now you are probably wondering why I eat so much grass-fed beef. There is a scientific explanation why fat from grass-fed cows helps you lose fat. Conjugated linoleic acid (CLA), is a fatty acid that's been proven by scientific studies to fight cancer, diabetes and reduce body fat.

Studies have also shown that CLA appears to reduce body fat while preserving muscle tissue, and the compound has become a huge boon to the supplement market, popular with bodybuilders and dieters. When found in a supplement form however, CLA is not in its natural balance so it is not without side effects. It is not nearly as effective as the CLA found naturally in grass-fed animals either.

I also want to address the issue of "fat farms" in this section because it fits right in with the crash diet schemes. Most camps, retreats or weight loss ranches promote lots of activity and very restricted calories to lose weight fast. The program is designed for muscle loss and water loss mainly, so the customers see lots of scale movement in a short period of time. People see this as success and end up coming back every year to lose the same 15 pounds over and over.

When they go back home, the weight comes back on and more, with less muscle to fight off new fat gain, so they are much worse off. After repeating this cycle for a few years, their metabolism is shot and so is their bank account. Quick weight loss is never a good idea, no matter where you are or how you do it. The body can change rapidly, but the mind usually takes more time, and both have to change together for permanent transformation to occur.

CHAPTER ELEVEN

CRACKING YOUR TRAVEL NUTRITION CODE

Proper nutrition at home is one thing. That is much easier because you have got the grocery stores you are used to as well as your own fridge, pots, pans, and supplies. Once you are away from home, it is usually a much different story. Most of my clients travel often and must eat out with others for business meetings. I get asked at least once a week by someone how they can maintain a healthy nutrition style when eating out and on the road.

The simplest answer is steamed meat and veggies. Most restaurants can prepare some grilled or broiled white meat and steamed green veggies, even if it is not on their menu. That is actually easier for the cook to prepare than their regular menu items, so no one will be too inconvenienced by the request.

The chef will naturally want to cook everything in oil or butter so asking them to keep this out will help too. One of my clients got so fed up with chefs not honoring this request, she actually started telling the waiter the she was allergic to linoleic acid (the main in gradient in fat) and if the chef put any fat in her meal, she would need an epinephrine shot and CPR. They always got it right after that explanation!

Meat and veggies aren't always a realistic answer in every case though. If you are trying to close a deal over dinner and your guest is obese, eating steamed veggies and meat might make them feel uncomfortable. In that case, try ordering the healthiest thing possible from the menu and eat the protein and greens first. Then take your time with the rest and do most of the talking instead of eating. Drink tons of water so you stay looking busy with the meal. By the time you are done talking, the waiter has come by and cleared your plate, taking the "bad" food away. Now it is out of sight and no longer an issue.

Treat alcohol the same way. Pick up your glass often and just touch it to your lips without drinking any. Take a small sip every 5 times you do this so the level changes slowly in your glass. Your guest will perceive you are drinking just as much as they are, but after their 3rd glass, you aren't even half done with yours.

When you are by yourself on your trip, go to the grocery store for lunch instead of a restaurant. Buy meats, cheese, veggies, and check the refrigerated section for boiled eggs and high protein/low carb options to satisfy your hunger. I bring my protein powder and hand blender with me on trips to mix a quick shake when I can't find good restaurant options or grocery stores nearby.

Buffets are also a great way to eat well on a trip. I go to Vegas 1-2 times a year for fun or a fitness convention and have no trouble eating right at the many buffets in town. I just load up my plate with protein and green veggies to my heart's content. Sure, they put more fat in the food than I do at home, but as long as the carbs aren't there, that fat won't be stored.

Bring healthy snacks on the airplane to eat instead of the food they serve. Airplane meals and snacks are some of the least healthy foods on the planet. Their food needs a long shelf life so it is all heat-treated and stuffed with preservatives, salt and HFCS. Be sure to drink 8 oz. of water for every hour you are flying too, because the dry recirculated air will dehydrate you as well and make you more likely to become ill from someone else's virus or bacterial infection.

There are things you can buy in the store when you get into a pinch. I went through a local Safeway and put together the following list within 5 minutes of walking the aisles. If I can do this in 5 minutes, just think what you can come up with by taking a little bit of time and reading some labels!

1.) "Eating Right" brand beef barley soup
2.) Blueberries and lowfat cottage cheese
3.) Pre-chopped veggies
4.) Pre-made garden salad with meat and cheese and balsamic vinaigrette
5.) Kraft "Live Active" cheese snacks
6.) Light string cheese
7.) Valley Fresh 100% natural white chicken bag
8.) Bumble Bee chicken breast bag or pink salmon steak bag
9.) Chicken of the Sea salmon bag
10.) "Organics" sliced turkey breast and "Organics" sliced cheese (roll them together for a snack)
11.) Hard boiled eggs

CHAPTER TWELVE

CRACKING YOUR METABOLIC CODE

Your metabolic rate is made up the following factors: How high you believe your metabolism is; what you eat and when you eat it; how much muscle you have; what kind of muscle that is; and your family genetics. I listed these factors in order of significance because your attitude about your own metabolism is the biggest factor and your genetics is the smallest factor. All factors including genetics can be changed, so the metabolism you were born with is certainly not the metabolism you will die with or pass down to your kids.

Putting all these factors together and figuring them out for your specific metabolism is the key. It's also easier than you think. Your individual metabolic code is very different from other people's codes. What makes them burn fat might not work for you and vice versa.

You may also discover that when you find a plan that does work for you, that plan might only work for a while until a plateau sets in. In any case, once you have cracked your metabolic code you will know what does work best and how to modify it accordingly to stay lean, fit, and healthy for life.

Through extensive study and investigation into the latest scientific research, I have cracked the metabolic code and will explain to you why your diet and exercise programs aren't working, and even if they are, why they are taking so much time and effort!

CRACKING YOUR FAT BURNING CODE

We all know at least a few people who can eat anything they want and never gain an ounce. We tend to have jealous thoughts toward them, but the reality is that they are probably just a natural fat burner. Their usual explanation is that they just have a "high metabolism" but it is their TYPE of metabolism that makes the difference.

There are two main categories of metabolisms. Most people are either a fat burner or a sugar burner. If you are a sugar burner you probably have a harder time getting lean and staying lean. You may actually have a higher metabolism and burn more calories than the skinnier fat burner you envy, but it is your type that makes the difference.

When I talk about sugar, I'm not just referring to table sugar (sucrose). While that is of course a sugar, it is only one kind. Sugar comes in many forms ranging from fast sugar like sucrose to slow sugar foods like the kind found in broccoli. Sucrose is a carbohydrate just like broccoli, but the structure of the carbohydrate is very different. These structure variations have different effects on your metabolism and must be understood completely to crack your metabolic code.

If you are a sugar burner, it just means your primary fuel source comes from carbohydrates, and fat is more easily stored. If you are a fat burner, it means you have an easier time liberating fat from your tissues and you also tend to burn fat as your primary energy source. I have a machine that measures this difference and tells clients what kind of burner they are, so I have seen all types. Most people are a combination of both, but I have tested some extremes as high as 95% one way or the other.

Recent scientific discoveries prove that not all metabolisms are the same, and some adjust up and down more than others. It's not fair that some of us are born sugar burners and others fat burners, but the good news is that you can modify your burn ratio and eventually teach your body to switch over.

Becoming a fat burner is of course the goal. Natural sugar burners do have to work harder at this transformation. Sugar burners also have deeper cravings for fat storing foods, so discipline is more of a factor, but if it is taken step by step, switching over to being a fat burner is a very realistic goal, even for the staunchest sugar burner.

A fat burner's metabolism also tends to be more dynamic than a sugar burner's. It will adjust up easier for a higher food intake and will even make the person "hot and sweaty" after a big meal like Thanksgiving dinner. The sugar burner might not feel this effect, and may even get colder after a meal.

The hard-core fat burners don't usually have the cravings that can turn them into sugar burners, so staying a fat burner often takes care of itself. This isn't fair either, but the good news to sugar burners is that converting into a fat burner is very doable with consistency and commitment. The time required to convert will depend on your present state (how much of a sugar burner you are), and how long you have been that way. If you have been a 95 percent sugar burner for 50 years it won't happen overnight, but it is still possible.

Fat burners can follow these same guidelines to remain as you are. These guidelines will also help ingrain it further into your metabolism and make you more resistant to turning into a sugar burner later.

If you reduce the fast sugar foods in your diet you will wean your body of this as its primary fuel source. If you are a hard-core sugar burner you probably crave carbs almost as much as the air you breathe, so reducing them will be tough if you try to take steps that are too large.

Never refuse yourself a food completely. Cutting something out of your diet will only make you crave it more, and may even cause you to obsess over it. This will result in failure and then abandonment because it will play with your mind too much and make your craving even stronger by grooving your brain pathways deeper over time.

For the strong sugar cravings, migrate your consumption of those foods to the middle of the day. This is a very high metabolic time, so your body will find it easier to burn it off and will be less likely to store it. Review the EFT chapter earlier in this book to help you break the uncontrollable cravings. Combining that skill with the mental techniques in this book will prove to be the one-two punch to knock the cravings out for good.

Exercise is an important step as well, because your internal health is dependent on your internal fitness. Exercise is listed as the last two steps in a seven step process to become a fat burner because nutrition is more important, but they must both go together for you to be truly successful as a permanent fat burner.

These seven steps should be followed in order because some complement others, and the progression makes it much easier to master. Be patient in completing each step and make sure you do so carefully and diligently.

Fat burner conversion step number one: Crank up Your Sleeping Fat Furnace

We spend about one third or our life sleeping. Normally, the metabolism declines steadily as the night progresses because our energy output is reduced and we get further and further into a fasted state as the hours go by. Most people eat comfort food and drink alcohol in the evening which drastically encourages fat storing even more. This habit causes most Americans to wake up fatter than when they went to bed!

Sleeping doesn't have to be wasted time or a fat gaining experience. It can be quite the opposite and used to your advantage as a time to burn fat off of your body instead. Your body will always burn a mixture of fat and carbs. As you sleep and run low on fuel (because you are not eating), your fuel burn mixture shifts more into fat burning mode and away from carb burning mode through the night.

When you are in your fat burning mode during the day, you might notice you are hungry or even tired. This can be unpleasant, but if you are asleep, you won't notice either of these issues. Taking advantage of your sleep time and making it work for you can make all the difference in the world for your fat burning goals.

Your first step should be to allow yourself only white meat, green vegetables and water after 7 pm. This sets your body up to be a fat burning furnace while you sleep. When this becomes easy, bump the cutoff point back to six pm, then five pm, and so on all the way until 2 pm, being careful to progress in steps only when you are ready.

Here's how it works: your body will run on carbs if they are provided. If carbs are taken away, it is forced into changing its fuel burn mixture to include more fat. With a carb cutoff time, your body has already begun to turn this direction when bedtime comes, and it progresses even further as you sleep. Being in a fat burning mode makes most of us hungry (which isn't too much fun) so what better time for that than when you're asleep and don't know it?

White meat has no carbs and is very low fat. White meat also has a very high metabolic cost. Your body will not want to convert it into fat or carbs because it's just too much trouble. It prefers to simply crank up its own metabolism instead, and just burn it off.

Fat doesn't need conversion. It's already fat. Carbs have to be converted to fat, and this takes energy, so some of the carbs are burned off in the conversion process. Complex carbs take more work than sugar carbs, and high fructose corn syrup takes little to no work of all. Protein on the other hand, is rarely converted into fat because it takes more energy for the body to do that than to just burn it off. Since the body will always choose the most efficient route, it will usually just raise its own metabolism to burn off the types of calories that are hard to convert.

Dark greens have the same metabolic cost. They also make your body think it's getting carbs and actually trick it into switching into the fat burning zone earlier than it would otherwise. The abundant nutrients in dark greens meet the body's vitamin quotas as well, so it knows it's getting proper nutrition and will not switch over into the dreaded "starvation mode" which tanks your metabolism.

If you are skeptical, just try it out. Chow down as much white meat and broccoli as you can eat and see what happens. After about 20-40 minutes you will feel like someone turned the thermostat up in your house. You will also feel an energy increase. This is your metabolism taking the easy way out by burning it off instead of converting it to fat.

Eating these foods in the evening helps put your body in its fat burning mode all night while you sleep, making valuable use of this time. This metabolism elevation, along with the improved fat fuel mixture burn, will turn you into a fat burning machine the whole time you sleep. Sawing logs is now productive time instead of wasted time!

I know some of you hate greens. I used to as well, but now crave them like I used to crave candy. Steamed broccoli and Tilapia fish with some curry powder and sea salt is all I need to go to bed happy and content. It sure didn't used to be like that though. I never liked non-fat milk either, but now it's the only kind I do like. If you introduce these foods in small steps, you will acquire the taste and it will only get easier.

People laugh at me when I tell them my favorite dessert is broiled broccoli with sea salt, but when they try it, they are instant converts. Little tricks found through experimentation produce great snippets that turn into gems when it comes to finding your own treats. My kids now beg for my broiled broccoli, and they still hate veggies! See the recipe section for this easy snack.

People acquire tastes all the time. Beer, wine, and cigars are all pretty nasty the first time out, but after a while they become pleasant and even craved. If people can force themselves into liking those bad habits, broccoli or kale certainly isn't a stretch! Your body will help you develop cravings for healthy foods because it knows they are good for your cells and help repair and build the whole system.

Steaming your foods will keep the moisture in and help with flavor. Few people enjoy raw greens, but five minutes of steam makes them a whole different story. The same goes for fish. Don't worry, if you detest fish you don't have to force yourself. There are plenty of other white meats out there that are just as good.

Spices are also encouraged as long as they don't possess any carbs. Base dry spices like pepper, curry, etc. are best. Adding peppers and spices to your food will elevate your metabolism without adding fat or carbs as a fuel source.

Salt is OK too if you don't have a blood pressure problem. Put spices on before you steam so they can cook into the food, but wait until after steaming to add the salt. This way you will use less and taste it more. Most sauces, marinades, and seasoning liquids are too high in carbs or fat, so steer clear of these unless the label says otherwise.

This plan allows you to "cheat" during the day. For this first step just make sure you are perfect after 7 pm. If you crave certain foods (and you will), just tell yourself you only have to wait until tomorrow to have it, and think about the foods you should be eating next. That will reduce the discipline requirement to a reasonable level.

When you master the 7 pm cutoff time, bump it to 6 pm, and then to 5 pm when you are ready. When you master the 5 pm cutoff time, step one is complete. Keep moving the cutoff to 2 pm, but when you do reach the 5 pm cutoff, you can move to step 2.

Remember to practice the technique from the beginning of this book about focusing on what you should be eating instead of what you will eat at your "cheat" period. Focusing on the healthy foods you want to start craving will help you trend toward those foods, and will weaken your cravings for the foods you want to stop craving. Thinking too much about the foods you will "cheat" with will only make cravings for those foods stronger, and will keep you in this stage longer than necessary.

If you must eat late at night, choose cottage cheese as a late night snack. If you get the late night munchies, go for some nonfat cottage cheese. This food releases slowly and keeps your fat furnace burning through the night. It also has a protein buffering effect which will help preserve muscle through the night better than other protein sources.

This nutrient timing is a very important habit to develop. Your metabolism will adjust up and down during the day depending on what you eat, when you eat it, your mood, stress levels, daily activity, and even sleep patterns. This is why a dietician can prescribe a certain number of calories and then watch their patient gain weight instead of lose it. The assumption is that the patient is cheating or being dishonest, but either way despair quickly follows and then abandonment of the whole idea often results.

Drink cold water before bed. Your body will have to warm it up and will expend energy to do it. Since you are now burning more fat calories and you just took in none, your net will be negative fat loss.

Water before bed will also hydrate you so your liver can liberate the fat from your tissues as you sleep. You might find yourself getting up at night to take a bathroom trip, but just think, "Is it more inconvenient to get up at night or to be fat all day, every day?"

Do high intensity exercise in the evening. High intensity exercise (HIT) has a metabolic elevation of three to four hours after you are done, so fitting in a 20 minute evening session can raise your sleeping metabolic rate considerably. You have to try it out for yourself though, because some people find it harder to get to sleep if high intensity training is part of their evening routine, while others find it helpful. I have found that HIT cardio helps me get to sleep but HIT strength training keeps me up.

Be sure to get enough sleep. Getting too little sleep causes release of cortisol and other chemicals that encourage fat storage and muscle breakdown. Most research suggests 7-8 hours for optimal hormone balance and recovery.

Gain more muscle. Since your muscle mass is your metabolism, having more of it on you will help you burn more fat all day and all night. As mentioned earlier, the best type of muscle for burning fat is fast twitch fibers, and the best way to gain this type of muscle is of course through the strength and cardio methods in this book!

Fat burner conversion step number two: Water Water Everywhere

After you have mastered step one, you can start drinking more water to stoke your fat burning furnace. Making water a habit can be a challenge, but there are plenty of techniques to help you. It is easiest to master if you use the same bottle and refill it. Figure out how much it holds and stick with that. Under counting and over counting is much too easy without a known volume to refill.

The average American spends more than 200 hours of their life every year commuting to and from work. Why not use this time to hydrate? A new study, published by the American Journal of Preventive Medicine shows a strong link between time spent driving and obesity—every additional 30 minutes a person spends in a car translates into a three per cent greater chance of becoming obese.

Hydrating is one of the most important ways to prevent and reverse weight gain, so simply bringing water with you in the car so you can drink it on your way somewhere is a very easy way to crank up your water habit.

Another thing you can do is to have water with you at work so it is always by your side. When out and about, never pass a drinking fountain without stopping off and taking at least seven swallows. These are only a couple of easy suggestions. You will develop your own techniques too as you master this step.

If you forget however, don't guzzle all your water at once to catch up. Just drink a glass and start over. You won't be able to absorb more than 20 ounces per hour anyway, so spread it out through the whole day.

You will probably find yourself beating a path to the bathroom at first. This is because your body is used to being dehydrated, so it thinks the extra water is unnecessary. It doesn't know how to absorb or process it properly, but this too will pass and your body will turn around and crave it as your thirst mechanism finally starts working properly.

If you find yourself annoyed by the increase in bathroom trips, just ask the question, "What is more inconvenient, spending a little more time each day in the bathroom or being overweight all day every day?"

Your individual quota for the day can be easily calculated. Just take your bodyweight in pounds and drink half that amount in water ounces. If you weigh 200 pounds, you need a minimum of 100 ounces per day.

Hudor, the Miracle Substance

Have you heard of Hudor? Its effects overshadow even the most potent ancient Chinese herbs. Its healing capabilities outperform wonder drugs from deep in the Amazonian rain forest. It holds the key to countless health benefits and wellness miracles.

Hudor can make your nails stronger, hair healthier, and teeth whiter. It greatly reduces skin problems and acne. It can even take away wrinkles and make your lips fuller. It promotes better skin circulation and tone, while often adding color as well. Hudor can heal chapped lips and dry mouth. Even chronic bad breath is often neutralized with proper doses.

Hudor acts as a catalyst for transporting essential nutrients throughout the body and performs as a solvent for all products of digestion, aiding the absorption through the intestinal walls into the bloodstream.

Hudor promotes protein metabolism better than anabolic steroids. It also metabolizes energy-producing carbohydrates. It prevents muscle cramping, increases physical performance, strength and endurance, and can lower your pulse rate and blood pressure. It is the best substance for maintaining electrolyte balance. It is the only proven ergogenic aid with no side effects or restrictions from the Food and Drug Administration.

The minerals potassium, sodium, magnesium, and calcium are essential for conducting electrical currents from the brain to the nervous system, and then to the muscles signaling contractions. Hudor promotes this more effectively than any other element even to the extent of preventing heart attacks.

Hudor also removes waste products from the body while simultaneously regulating its temperature. It is the key ingredient in chemical reactions that metabolize stored fat—especially when taken just before a meal and again right after. It can also act as a potent appetite suppressant, filling you up without any chemical side effects.

It promotes healing of injuries as well as illness. It boosts the immune system's defenses better than any drug on the market. It holds the key to transporting antioxidants and aids in their effectiveness to fight cancer. It improves general comfort, mood, and well being, while decreasing irritability and nervousness. It helps prevent fatigue and improves concentration, memory, and alertness.

Cuts, bruises and even tendonitis are healed up to twice as fast with proper amounts of Hudor, and chronic daily headaches are often permanently cured. Muscle soreness from injury, overuse or exercise is cut in half or less with Hudor. It also lengthens the life of all vital organs-especially the liver and kidneys, and is still available over the counter!

The significance of the liver and kidney health is especially important to fat loss. If the kidneys are functioning properly, the liver doesn't have to help them out and can concentrate on its job of taking fat out of your tissues to be burned off. Hudor directly affects both kidney and liver health in a very specific way which in turn accelerates fat loss.

Where do you get Hudor? It has been around since before man existed. Your body is made up of 65 percent Hudor. It takes up more than 70 percent of the earth's surface, and the nearest source is your tap. Hudor is the Greek word for water and you're probably not getting enough.

The average person loses two cups of water through normal perspiration. Another two cups is exhaled as water vapor during the process of breathing. Together, the intestines and kidneys use about four cups a day. That's eight cups used just for living, not counting anything extra we might do during the day.

*If you drink at least three quarts or more a day you're already experiencing its wonderful effects. If you are like most Americans who drink dehydrating beverages like coffee, soda and alcohol with very little water, the effects of three quarts or more daily will truly be miraculous. You may find yourself in the restroom more frequently, but just ask yourself, which is more inconvenient: finding a bathroom more often or carrying around extra weight and being less healthy **all** the time?*

Make sure you're drinking it plain too. Mineral and sparkling water often contain too much sodium. Soft drinks are even worse. Although their main ingredient is water, less than ten percent of it will be absorbed because of all the preservatives, dyes, flavoring agents, sugar, sodium, and additives.

Pure, clean water is absorbed through the lining of the intestines. Juice, coffee, or soda is held within the intestines for further digestion. The process of digesting these other drinks can require even more water than originally found in the beverage! These drinks may further encourage dehydration, rather than relieving it. Try to get filtered water whenever possible. Reverse osmosis systems are the most effective at taking out the harmful chemicals, indigestible minerals, and sediment often found in municipal sources.

If additional water is not consumed to make up for a deficit, the body may be forced to draw upon itself from the areas of richest supply; namely the muscles. When muscle tissue dehydrates by even as little as three percent, it will lose ten percent of its contractile strength and eight percent of its speed. Dehydration also adversely affects the structure and function of the nervous system, producing a miniscule but crucial shrinkage of the brain resulting in decreased concentration, coordination, performance, and headaches.

To obtain the benefits of the wonder fluid, go straight to the source and get the real thing in its cleanest form. The next time you find it hard to move off the couch, can't concentrate, or are having a bad day; pour yourself a big glass of filtered water. It may also be the key to losing those last few stubborn pounds or the cure to a frustrating fitness plateau. It's worth a try. It may be just that simple.

I wrote this Hudor article back in 1990 for the clients I didn't seem to be getting through to about water. They always asked me about the latest diet craze or supplement pill, but when I asked them about their water intake, the answer was usually, "I'm trying" which in other words means, "I really haven't given it much effort."

I decided to write an article like the supplement companies do, using the same buzz words and psychological tactics. It worked too. Half way through the article, my clients couldn't wait to get a hold of Hudor and wondered why I finally "sold out" to promote a particular supplement. Then when they got the end, they just laughed and said, "OK I get it now, I'll start drinking my water."

I have also been approached occasionally by hydration naysayers who claim we really don't need all this water. In fact, they claim we don't even need the 8 glass per day recommendation most nutritionists prescribe. This is a pet peeve of mine so please allow me to go on a rant here.

I feel that proper hydration is the single most important ingredient in any fitness program and is absolutely vital for good health, so I am more passionate about this topic than any other. If you sense the tone of this book changing through the next few pages, you are picking up on my anger towards the incompetent individuals who recommend less than 8 glasses per day!

I feel that 8 glasses per day is actually not enough for most people. I'm really irritated with a few quacks ("Dorkters" I like to call them) blithering on about how we don't really need to drink 8 glasses of water per day. They are just trying to get press time and create a stir by going against current wisdom and sound, healthy advice.

The interesting fact to me, is that these Dorkters don't cite any reasons that drinking 8 glasses of water is bad! They make the false claim that there aren't enough well designed research studies proving 8 glasses or more is necessary, but totally neglect to cite a single study that supports drinking less than 8 glasses a day. It took me all of about 10 minutes to find over a dozen research studies to support my opinion. Anyone can Google *Pub Med Online* and see for them self how many well designed studies are out there now.

Shouldn't doctors be spending their time telling us about stuff that would harm us or help us, instead of wasting their time talking about stuff that doesn't matter if it isn't true? This just proves my point that they are pointlessly blithering because they know it will get them some attention. There are no health problems associated with drinking 8 glasses per day, but many serious health problems have been proven to result from drinking less than 8 glasses a day, including death! Shouldn't the Dorkters err on the safe side if they are doing us a service and not try to convert people to hypo hydration and all of its proven risks?

So far every "expert" I have seen who has claimed that we d
8 or more glasses of water per day has a little fat to lose themse\
every layperson who has repeated this message to me has also ueen at
least moderately overweight. If I am only hearing this message from those
with excess weight, it sure seems to confirm the fat loss benefits of proper
hydration.

I did run across one water-naysayer who appeared to be relatively thin
(at least between the ears), but I could detect a little "pooch" in his stomach
area despite his loose shirt. He stated he was proof that my claim in the
preceding paragraph was false, so I just responded, "OK, I'll count to three,
and then we will both pull up our shirts and do a quick comparison of my
12-20 cups a day abs to your 5-7 cups a day abs." I started counting, and
by the time I got to 2, he had already turned around and stormed off.

Our brains are 85% water, so it figures that only the dehydrated people
are preaching the less water message in spite of all the scientific evidence
available. Even if there were no scientific proof for proper hydration, it
would still make for basic common sense. I guess us smart, hydrated folks
have to "dumb it down" for the dehydrated population.

With the lack of water intake, abundance of coffee, sodas, and alcohol,
it's no wonder everyone is always sick and overweight! The bottom line
is that even if you doubt what I am saying here, the risk of getting too
little water is much worse than the risk of getting a little too much. If I'm
wrong, you are only making more trips the bathroom. If I'm right, your
whole life changes, and I've seen that happen over and over! Let's just
look at a few of the most common general knowledge side effects of both
sides of the coin:

Problems With Chronic Dehydration	Problems with Slight Over hydration
Slow to no fat los	More trips to the bathroom
Kidney stones	
Headaches	
Decreased strength	
Decreased concentration	
Muscle cramps	
Indigestion	
Heart problems	
Liver problems	
Elevated blood pressure	

Irregular body temperature
More frequent illnesses
45 to 79% increased cancer risk
Joint pain
Vertebral disk degeneration
Sodium retention
Water retention
Bad breath
Gallstones
Urinary tract infections
Gout
Osteoporosis
Skin problems/acne
More skin wrinkles
Chapped lips
Decreased circulation
Intestinal problems
Decreased endurance
Increased appetite
Slower healing and repair
Increased muscle soreness
Mood swings
Hormone regulation problems
Eyesight degeneration
Slower metabolism

The low-water "Dorkters" also waste their time talking about the dangers of drastic over hydration. Drinking too much water to the point of upsetting your electrolyte balance (hyponatremia) is very hard to do. This would require drinking at least your weight in ounces over a 12 hour period, so hyponatremia really isn't an issue for people without Obsessive Compulsive Disorder. Some extreme endurance athletes and babies of stupid parents can fall victim to hyponatremia, but it takes such high water volumes to cause problems (especially in our high sodium culture), it's hardly worth mentioning.

If you want to know how much water your body uses in a day, just weigh yourself right before bed, and then again right when you wake up. You will be 1-2 pounds lighter in the morning, simply from exhaling water vapor while you slept! This means that if you stayed asleep for 24 hours, you would breathe out 48-96 ounces of water in that time. This equates to 6-12 glasses of water right there! Now add normal daily activities with some conversation, and you are already over the traditional 8 glass recommendation even before exercise!

Our thirst mechanisms do not work right when we are chronically dehydrated. Our bodies are forced to pull water out of our food to keep us alive, and this teaches our system to tell us we are *hungry* when we are really just *thirsty*! Dehydrated people have taught their bodies that it must get its water from food, so it craves food instead of water when it really just needs water!

If you don't believe this, try drinking your proper amount of water for 3 weeks, and you will see for yourself that you get thirsty more often than you get hungry instead of vice versa. This is because when you are properly hydrated, and your body is getting its needs from water instead of extracting it from food, it just asks for more water! Many people have lost fat from proper hydration alone, because their food consumption goes down so much after their thirst mechanism gets dialed in properly.

Fat loss from proper hydration is also tied into your liver function. When you are dehydrated, your kidneys need help and your liver comes to their rescue. One of the liver's main jobs is to extract fat out of your tissues to be burned off, and when the liver is busy helping the kidneys, guess which job it's not doing anymore?

Water also keeps your immune system functioning optimally. When we are ill, we lose water at an accelerated rate because we are blowing our nose, sweating, coughing, expectorating, and in the worst cases, launching out one end and/or the other. Lots of fluid is being lost and it must be replenished quickly, because our cells are 70-90% water and this is where the war is waging between the good guys and the virus or bacteria!

Your blood plasma is mostly water. Plasma acts as a reservoir that can either replenish insufficient water or absorb excess water from tissues. When body tissues need additional liquid, water from plasma is the first resource to meet that need. Plasma circulation plays a vital role in regulating body temperature by carrying heat generated in core body tissues through areas that lose heat more readily, such as the arms, legs, and head. It's pretty easy to see the damage done when you are dehydrated while you are sick with a fever.

Your skin is your first defense against infection. When you are dehydrated, your skin cracks and your lips chap. This provides nice little gateways for tiny little viruses and bacteria to sneak through. Mucus membranes are also one of your first lines of defense. When those are dried up from a lack of water, bad stuff gets by them too. White blood cells are the internal defense mechanisms that take care of the stuff that gets into your bloodstream. Guess what their main ingredient is? Yep, water. They can't fight for you effectively if you are not hydrating them too!

Another reason I preach water so hard is because your muscles are 75% water. When you exercise, you are breaking down your muscles, much like a tornado would break down your house. If you give your body a little excess water, you are providing excess building materials to rebuild it stronger than before. This is like Home Depot dropping off too much lumber to rebuild your house after the storm. You get to add on and make it better!

The only way you can depend on your thirst mechanism to accurately tell you when you need water (and not more food) is to be properly hydrated. To calculate your water needs, divide your body weight in half and then drink that many ounces of water each day. Some people under 100 pounds might need more, and others over 250 pounds might need less, but it's a good general rule.

Another important point the Dorkters fail to mention is that heavy people, well-muscled individuals, and genetically heavy sweaters will suffer much worse effects from less than 8 glasses a day than those of "normal weight" and sweat rates. Under-hydrated individuals with weight problems will crave food to satisfy their broken thirst mechanism even more than normal weight people, which further perpetuates their weight problem.

Children are at greater risk for dehydration than adults due to their higher surface-to-mass ratio. Additionally, children have different thirst sensitivities and body cooling mechanisms than adults. Children differ from adults in total body water content, and boys and girls differ in body water content with maturation. Research in young adults shows that mild dehydration corresponding to only 1% to 2% of body weight loss can lead to significant impairment in cognitive function. Dehydration in infants is associated with confusion, irritability, and lethargy; in children, it even produces decrements in cognitive performance.

The research makes the case for proper hydration indisputable, and simple common sense verifies it. Water is free, so I'm not getting anything out of being on this soap box other than the satisfaction of seeing you succeed in your fitness and health goals. Just do it!

Fat burner conversion step number three: Protein Quotas

Once you master step two, make sure you are getting enough protein before 5 pm as well. You can still eat whatever you want before five pm, but it has to include 80 grams of protein if you are a woman or 100 grams of protein if you are a man.

Following labels and keeping a running tally is too confusing, not to mention too much work! There is an easier way and it just means eating four servings of meat as big as your fist. It works just the same whether you are a man or woman, because men usually have bigger fists so they will get more protein.

Larger framed men and women will also need more protein too, so that is another way the fist measuring technique works well. You can, of course, get protein from vegetarian sources as well, so in that case you may have to resort to reading labels, but to keep it as simple as possible, stick with meat whenever you can.

Organic meat is the best because non-organic varieties can have harmful chemicals and hormones that will interfere with your fat-burning metabolism. These toxins can even be stored in your fat tissues making it harder to lose the fat, and can increase cravings for that particular food later.

White meat is of course the lowest fat content, and wild white fish is the best because it is naturally organic. Big fish that live a long time however, can accumulate high levels of metals in their tissue that can slow the fat liberation process, so be careful where the fish comes from and how old it is.

You can do a quick search on your own using the internet to find out different estimated levels of metals in different fish and areas. This research is especially necessary for pregnant and lactating women, because while no one wants to build up levels in their own body, passing it on to baby is even worse since brain and other tissue development is so rapid at this time.

Grass-fed beef also works well for most people. Grass-fed is even better than organic beef because it has a certain kind of fat that encourages your metabolism to burn off your own body fat. This type of fat is called conjugated linoleic acid (CLA), and is found in the highest quantities and the right ratios almost exclusively in grass-fed animals. Big game animals other than cattle also have this type of fat. Grass-fed organic is of course the best, but many grass-fed farms use fertilizer to grow grass. While this fertilizer is harmless to you, it does kick them out of the organic qualification.

Vegetarians will have a harder time getting enough protein than meat-eaters. Soy is the only complete protein source so I encourage many strict vegetarians (vegans) to supplement with low fat/low carb soy sources or a soy powder protein shake. Since vegetarians also get higher levels of Omega 6 fatty acids than Omega 3, they might also need to supplement with Omega 3 oil to balance that back out.

Fat burner conversion step number four: Go to Your Roots

Now that we have talked about eating things with legs or fins, we should discuss the importance of eating things with roots. When you master your quotas for water and protein, you can move on to this fourth step. This step involves adding in two servings of vegetables and one serving of fruit before your cutoff time.

Each serving should be the size of your fist. You can still cheat with the foods you crave, but just make sure you give priority to your quotas of protein, water, fruit and vegetables first. Space them out through the day so you don't find yourself gorging your quotas at the last minute. Make Tupperware your best friend and take your quotas with you in the morning. A little planning ahead goes a long way and makes it so much easier.

Eating properly proportioned fiber foods can optimize fat burning as well. Fiber fills you up and many even believe it binds with fat to pull some out of your body. Most green vegetables have the proper fiber proportions built in, but there are other sources as well. I frequently enjoy a burrito when I have the hankering because I have found the perfect tortilla. With eleven grams of carbs and eight of them coming from fiber, it is quite a powerhouse for taste, fiber, and macronutrient ratios.

When you can do these four steps consistently you are on your way to becoming (or staying) a fat burner. There are even more advanced techniques later in this book for turning up your fat burning stove further, but these steps followed with consistency, will give you the metabolism you have always wanted.

This system will also teach you the importance of timing your macronutrients. You could eat the exact same thing but reverse the time of day and it won't work. If you eat your meat and veggies for lunch and cheat foods in the morning or at night, you will gain fat or find it hard to lose it at best.

When I tried this program on myself I gave it four months. It started out as an experiment to find a system to maintain my already low body fat level while allowing some "cheating." I would have been happy to just maintain my 10% body fat at the time, but I did actually lose more fat in spite of occasional Dove ice cream bars during the day and occasional lunch out!

When I switched over and cheated at night, I only lasted two weeks before I had to bail out because I was gaining weight so fast! *The only thing I changed was the timing of the foods.* I was eating the same foods and identical calories but just flipped the timing. I ate the greens and meat up until 5 pm and the other foods after 5 pm. The actual cheat hours per day were less but in spite of that, it took only two weeks to put on twice the fat I had lost in the previous four months!

Fat burner conversion step number five: Gain Lean to Stay Lean

Let's face the facts. Most of your fat burner conversion will be achieved through your nutrition. Most of your short term fat loss will also be attained through nutrition. Strength training and anaerobic cardio exercise is important too however, because the techniques here will help you become a fat burner faster and will help you stay there after you achieve it.

You must gain muscle to be a permanent fat burner. This doesn't mean you have to "bulk up" by any means. In fact, as you gain muscle and swap out fat, you will become smaller even if the scale doesn't show it. I have had many clients actually gain weight while they watch their pants practically fall off of them from going down in sizes. I even had one client go from a size 16 to a 9 and lose only 11 pounds on the scale!

Pound for pound, muscle takes only about ½ the space of fat, so you can see how the inches fall off when you trade those tissues. The human form also takes improved shape with added muscle. If you take a close look at an Olympic sprinter, you will see the fantastic form and shape muscle provides. This athlete however, will be as heavy or heavier on a scale than his or her sedentary counterpart of the same height who doesn't eat right or workout.

I am reminded how much people really do like the look of the track and field athletes every four years during the summer games. Women everywhere are always talking about the women sprinters and mid distance runners. For the next year, the covers of all the fitness magazines display these new Olympic champions.

Female runway models on the other hand, might look OK on the runway with the right lights, clothes, and enough layers of makeup, but if you saw them naked before their morning shower, your screams of disgust would be heard for miles. Their lack of muscle makes them look frail and downright unhealthy.

Curves are attractive, and the only way to put them where you want them is through the right exercise practices. You cannot spot reduce fat deposits or pick an area to slim down, but you can pick an area you want to add curves or shape to, and tone up with new muscle through exercise.

You can also sculpt your body to create visual illusions of thinness in areas you want by shaping others with exercise. If you have a broad waist for instance, you can build your back and shoulders in a way that makes your waist look smaller. Wide thighs can be "slimmed" through appearance by shaping the calves.

These are just a couple of examples of the many ways you can sculpt your body to create new proportions to achieve the look you have always wanted, no matter what frame or body type you were born with.

Whether you are gaining muscle to shape, reduce, or just affect your metabolism, you are contributing to your fat burning furnace. Every pound of muscle you add raises your fat burning metabolism all day, every day. It even causes you to burn more fat while you sleep simply by having muscle on your frame.

More muscle is the main reason men have higher metabolisms than women. Muscle loss is also the main reason our metabolism declines with age. If we add muscle, our metabolism goes up proportionally, and if we swap fat for muscle, it goes up even more.

Strength training is the best way to add muscle, and the section, "Cracking your strength code" is the best way to strength train. You will learn the quickest and safest way to trade fat for muscle and shape yourself the way you want to look faster than any other system out there. You can now benefit from what recent science has to say about exercise, instead of spinning your wheels with the outdated system everyone else uses.

Cardiovascular exercise burns fat immediately through the exercise itself, but how you do it will determine whether it sets you up as an ongoing fat furnace or just a quick spark. There are many different cardiovascular workouts, but very few that continue to work through the rest of your life.

How many long-time distance runners do you see who are skinny in places but still have fat "pockets" in others that never seem to go away? How many of those people look toned everywhere and have a desirable shape? I can't think of many. That's because long duration cardio exercise wastes muscle and takes away from shape and tone. It also stops working as a fat reducer after a while because the body becomes so efficient at it by adapting to the activity.

The die-hard aerobic folks will argue that metabolism is altered through the increased mitochondria count in the muscles. These little endurance engines within the muscle do indeed help you burn more calories, but when muscle is being reduced in mass through endurance exercise, their impact is also reduced.

Unless you are training for an endurance sport, you don't ever need to do endurance training. It is a colossal waste of time. You can get similar mitochondria count increases and build muscle at the same time with the anaerobic cardio methods in this book. Your metabolism will also increase over time instead of decline as with traditional cardio.

When I talk about anaerobic exercise I am referring to sprint training. As you perform sprints, you are using oxygen faster than your body can deliver it to the muscles, and through certain interval segment timing, you will set yourself up to burn about four times more fat than long duration cardio in about one third the time!

No effective exercise is easy, but there are certainly shorter and better ways. The best way to do cardio exercise is through the sprint intervals I'm talking about here. These short sprint segments create heart rate spikes that cause your metabolism to "freak out" after you are done, for up to twelve times the amount of time you spent doing the exercise itself!

Regular steady state aerobic cardio exercise elevates your post exercise metabolism for only about the same amount of time you spent in the exercise. In other words, if you go for an hour run, your metabolism will remain elevated for about an hour after you are done. A proper 20 minute sprint interval session as described later in the section "Cracking Your Cardio Code", will elevate your metabolism for three to four hours after you are done!

Recent research from the Boston University School of Medicine found that fast twitch muscle fibers raise your metabolism more than slow twitch fibers. If you took an endurance runner with mostly slow twitch fibers, and compared their metabolism to a strength trainer with fast twitch fiber of the same body weight, the strength trainer would have the higher metabolism.

The endurance runner would burn more calories through exercise each day because they are training much more than the strength trainer, but the strength trainer would burn more calories doing nothing and while sleeping. More of those calories burned are from fat on the strength trainer as well. Sprint training and strength training following the methods in this book will emphasize your fast twitch fibers and maximize this metabolic elevation.

Fat burner conversion step number six: Phasing into Grazing

Break up your meals into small segments so you are eating many times through the day. You have heard many recent experts tell you to eat five to six meals a day instead of the traditional three, but you can take that a step further by breaking your meals up into even smaller pieces and grazing all day. I eat in the car, at my computer, at work, and spread it out all day long.

The timing of your macronutrients is another important component in your fat burning formula. If you eat protein in the morning and low carbs, you are continuing your fat burning zone from last night. Eating fiber at your afternoon snack will make you less hungry at dinnertime. These are only a couple of recommendations for food type timing. For a winning macronutrient combination example, try the following:

Breakfast:
- 20 oz. water
- Egg white omelet with spinach, and lean meat (see the "*PJoe's Special*" recipe in the chapter "Cracking Your Recipe Code) OR natural protein shake (protein powder sweetened with Stevia and organic milk or organic soy milk).

Mid-morning snack:
- 16 oz. water
- Any dark green vegetable and lean meat

Lunch:
- 20 oz. water
- Mixed green salad with chicken and oil-free balsamic dressing OR high fiber meat wrap (see Fiberilla Burrito in the recipe chapter).

Afternoon snack:
- 16 oz. water
- Any dark green vegetable and lean meat

Dinner:
- 20 oz. water
- Roasted green veggies
- Spicy Peanut Bake (see recipe chapter) OR lean meat

Night time snack:
- 16 oz. water
- Any dark green vegetable and lean meat OR lowfat cottage cheese

Notice that I didn't give any amount restrictions or portion recommendations on these foods. This is because everyone is different and these foods can be eaten in any amount. If you eat more at one time of day however, you will naturally eat less at the next meal, so it all evens itself out anyway.

Fat burner conversion step number seven: Teetotalers Rule the World

Wean yourself off alcohol. I know I lost many of you with this one! Your emotions may have dropped, and your anxiety increased, but don't worry! With the techniques in the first section and the EFT method in chapter eight, you can get rid of this issue as well—even if you don't want to!

I have talked to dozens of people who all say the same thing, "I will do anything you say but please don't take away my drink. It is the only vice I have left and I will not part with it." Eventually those people not only stop drinking alcohol, they can't believe they ever said that either!

Let me explain how alcohol stops your fat burning process. I know this topic is revisited at other points in this book, but only because it is that important to understand. If you get tired of reading my "repeated explanations," just know there is a method to this madness as well. I am drilling certain pertinent points into your subconscious so it gets the message even before your conscious mind does. Since your subconscious will control whether you crave alcohol or not, this is very important.

Alcohol is a very unique calorie. Each gram holds 7 calories but acts totally different from other types of calories. Carbs and protein hold 4 calories per gram and fat holds 9 calories per gram. Protein, carbs, and fat all increase your metabolism (in the order I listed them), and they all encourage you to burn a mixed fuel source of carbs, fat and protein (in that order as well).

Alcohol on the other hand, will cause your body to run almost exclusively on it as a fuel source until it is out of your bloodstream. Little to no fat burning or carb burning is taking place. This goes on proportionally to how many drinks you have, but most people can count on an hour for each drink for this fuel source to be burned away.

Only a small portion of the alcohol is converted into fat, but your liver then converts most of the alcohol into acetate. The acetate is then released into your bloodstream, and *replaces* fat as a source of fuel.

Not only does too much alcohol put the brakes on fat burning, it's one of the most effective ways to slash your testosterone levels as well. Science has shown that just a single bout of heavy drinking raises levels of the muscle-wasting hormone cortisol and increases the breakdown of testosterone for up to 24 hours.

The damaging effects of alcohol on testosterone are made even worse when you exercise before drinking, so the pickup game of basketball and beers afterwards is quite a nasty knockdown punch for testosterone levels.

The effect of alcohol on testosterone could be one reason that people who drink a lot carry less muscle. In fact, a 1993 study shows that alcoholic men have bigger waists and smaller muscles than non-drinkers.

Now if that's not bad enough, add to it the fact that alcohol dehydrates you as well. This dehydration causes a strain on your kidneys, which requires your liver to help them out. When your liver is helping them out, it is putting its other jobs on hold. Guess what one of the liver's main jobs is? It's liberating your fat cells and emptying them out to be burned off.

Appetite is also increased by consuming alcohol. Certain chemicals are released in your brain, and the alcohol itself causes hormonal changes that increase your cravings for carbs and fat. This causes you to eat these types of foods and guess what happens to them? Because you are running on alcohol as your primary fuel source, those foods can't be burned off. The fat ends up being stored in your cells and the carbs are converted to fat, which is then stored in your cells also.

We have all heard that alcohol is a depressant and it slows the reflexes, slurs the speech, and makes us do stupid things, but it is a depressant for your metabolism as well. Besides running on alcohol as fuel, this substance causes you to burn less calories while it is in your system.

Instead of burning 100 calories an hour, with 50% of that coming from fat like you normally would, you end up burning 80 calories an hour with 5% or less of that coming from fat. This continues as long as it is in your bloodstream, which could be quite a while if the drinks are strong enough and the volume is significant.

Alcohol is the single most effective fat storing machine and sugar burning drug available. It is the one substance that works in the opposite direction from your efforts toward becoming a fat burner. Alcohol teaches your system how to get better at burning sugar and storing fat. Over time with continued drinking, your body unlearns its fat burning techniques and learns better fat storing methods instead.

Alcohol increases visceral fat storage more than any other type of calorie. Visceral fat is the fat that is underneath your stomach muscle and surrounds your organs. This fat has also been associated with high risk of heart problems, so avoiding its accumulation is desirable, to say the least. The increase in visceral fat is most evident by the "beer gut" common with regular drinkers.

You will hear many health and fitness experts claim there is no way to spot reduce fat in a certain area, and while this is largely true, this would be the exception, because cutting out alcohol will lead to reduction in belly fat first.

This seven step nutrition plan will indeed work forever, but your mind will plateau after a while, so pick another program from this book when that happens to help you stay on the lifestyle wagon. Remember this is not an aggressive weight loss diet. This is a base plan for turning yourself into a fat burner over time with permanent lifestyle changes.

7 FOODS THAT WILL INCREASE YOUR METABOLISM

These seven foods can be eaten anytime, anywhere, and in any amount. Yes, indeed! This is good news for compulsive overeaters and those who don't seem to stop eating when they are full. These seven options will not make you gain fat, and some may even cause you to lose fat. When you have the hunger pangs, psychological or physical, just go to these foods and have at them. They are nature's only guilt-free calories!

Let's start with the best and work our way down. The top two are white meat and broccoli. I challenge anyone in the world—even those with thyroid or other metabolic disorders to try to get fat on these two foods.

By white meat I mean any meat that is pure white in color. This includes many fish as well as crab and shrimp. It also includes a few different fowl, but be careful because fowl also has dark meat. Egg whites also can be included in this category.

118 CRACKING YOUR METABOLIC CODE

Lean protein like white meat tends not to be burned, because the body prefers to use this macronutrient as a building block instead of an energy source. Eating protein will cause more fat and carbs to be burned than you just ate, so that makes it a negative fat food.

The reason protein has this negative fat effect is because it is a very high metabolic calorie, which means it costs more energy for your body to process it than the other calorie types. Fat doesn't cost much energy to process because it is already in a useable and storable state, and doesn't need converting. Carbs cost more energy than fat because they do need to be converted to be used as energy, and then converted again to be stored. Lean protein on the other hand, is hardest for the body to break down, and extremely hard to convert into anything else. This makes your body want to just use it for building tissues or burn it off through an increased metabolic rate.

Since your metabolic calorie fuel mixture is predominately a combination of fat and carbs, you will burn more of those types of calories than the protein calories. Since the lean protein is what caused this metabolic elevation and it contains no carbs and very little fat, you are burning more of the other types of calories, which makes the negative fat effect happen.

Broccoli is a true superfood. There are so many different vitamins and minerals in broccoli, a person could actually thrive on a diet of meat and broccoli only for the rest of their life. The only vitamin that might be lacking would be vitamin D, and since the skin manufactures it, this could be taken care of with about 10 minutes of sunshine each day.

Even if someone with a metabolism of 2,000 calories was to eat 4,000 calories in white meat and dark greens each day, I guarantee they would LOSE fat. A registered dietician going by their textbooks would tell you that person would gain approximately four pounds per week on this kind of diet. In reality however, this person would not only lose fat, it they might even gain some muscle at the same time!

I realize this is nutritional blasphemy in some circles, but not only is this based in recent proven scientific data, I have seen this firsthand over and over with others, and have had the same results myself. This type of diet will help cleanse your insides as well, because white meat doesn't "stick" to your blood vessels and dark greens are so high in fiber, the bad stuff gets dragged right out with them.

The number three food is celery. You can juice it, steam it, eat it raw, or anything else, and it will satisfy your crunchies and munchies. The fiber it holds will stave off hunger, and the water content will aid your hydration.

Fourth best is hot chili peppers. Gram for gram, they contain more vitamin C and A than many dark greens, and digesting them actually increases your metabolism. Researchers have also reported that hot chili peppers specifically boost your fat burning metabolism by aiding in the oxidation of fat.

Fifth is leafy greens like collard greens, kale and spinach. These nutrient-dense foods also contribute lots of fiber, which aids in pulling out fat and other things that might cause you to gain fat. These can be cooked many different ways, but the least amount of cooking is best to preserve the nutrient content.

Sixth is the tomato. Tomatoes are actually just red bags of water and antioxidants. The water content of a tomato is even higher than watermelon, and high amounts of lycopene offer huge health benefits. I often eat these in raw slices with salt or Mrs. Dash. It's a great snack by itself or a fantastic addition to many recipes. There is even some research that suggests the antioxidant properties in tomatoes increase with cooking, so don't worry about losing nutrients in preparation with this superfood.

Seventh is Beets. Their high levels of potassium, calcium, and antioxidants combined with a positive effect on the metabolism make this food a winner. They are also believed to be a powerful cleanser of the blood and kidneys. Some studies even show a reduction in blood pressure from beet juice.

Beets are quite potent however, so you can overdo it. Too high of a concentration (juicing too many at one time) can make you feel pretty weird and even in some cases, temporarily paralyze your vocal chords, so don't go too crazy here!

Most spices and seasonings can also be used with these foods for flavoring and taste. Meat should always be cooked, but the veggies are best raw. If you do cook your veggies, steam or broil them. My favorite preparation style is to broil greens with garlic and Mrs. Dash sprinkled on top.

7 FOODS THAT WILL SLOW YOUR METABOLISM

We have talked about the seven free foods that will cause you to lose weight by eating them, but as with everything in life, there are opposites too. It's not fair that many more foods will make you gain fat than lose fat, but the following seven are the worst. Start cutting back on these immediately, because for a truly healthy lifestyle you will want to remove them from your life as much as you can.

The number one fat-adding culprit is alcohol. See the previous step **"Fat burner conversion step number seven"** for specifics on why it works so hard against your fat burning goals.

Sugar wins the silver medal for adding fat to your body. Sugar is one of the best ingredients at spiking your insulin levels, which put you in a fat-storing mode. It is also a toxin to the immune system and effectively crowds vitamin C right out of your cells. Sugar is the main reason so many more people get sick over the holidays than any other time of year. It is also the main cause of holiday weight gain each year.

If you don't believe this, try cutting sugar out of your diet from October to January and see how well you stay. Viruses and bacteria will bounce off you from all directions. You will also notice your weight level off or even go down. This ingredient is basically poison to your body and has no health benefits whatsoever.

High fructose corn syrup (HFCS) is even worse that sugar. HFCS suppresses your immune system even more than sugar and causes a multitude of additional health problems. HFCS is now found in everything from soda to salad dressing, and has been noted by many experts as a major culprit in the current obesity epidemic.

Fructose from HFCS is NOT the same molecule that is in fruit or sugar. There is more than 35 years of scientific evidence of refined man-made high fructose corn syrup (HFCS) metabolizing straight to fat, UNLIKE the fructose molecule linked to a glucose molecule, found in regular sugar (sucrose), which is converted to blood glucose before converting to fat if it can't be used for energy (if it is consumed in excess).

Here are the undisputable facts we have learned from objective and proven scientific studies and research:

- Sucrose raises blood glucose and then crashes it below baseline, within 25 minutes of ingestion.
- HFCS converts to fat within 60 minutes of ingestion.
- Since 1980, HFCS dietary increases have paralleled the American actuarial curve on diabetes, cardiovascular disease, hypoglycemia, and obesity.
- The cheapest ingredient in the American food chain after water and salt is HFCS.

- Before 1970, HFCS did not exist. Today Americans eat more than 67 pounds per person each year.

Sugar and HFCS are the two main reasons so many people get sick during the holidays. Some people attribute this season of sicknesses to school starting and the kids bringing stuff home. Others blame it on the colder weather, but the real reason is that starting in September, when the stores put out the Halloween candy, we start gobbling the sugar and HFCS like there is no tomorrow.

HFCS and sugar both compete with certain vitamins to cross your cell membranes. The same mechanism that brings vitamin C into your cells, brings sugar in as well. Since sugar is consumed in much larger quantities than vitamins, guess which one wins? Sugar and HFCS effectively push valuable immune fighters right out of your cells!

Obese people can store up to 35% of the sugar they consume as energy which can later be converted to fat if not used. HFCS is most prevalent in diet foods, so you can see how people continue to get fat on these foods.

Elevated insulin levels from sugar and HFCS also increase your appetite and cause you to eat more. In one obesity study, subjects whose insulin levels were stimulated by drinking water sweetened with HFCS out-ate the control group *by over 500 calories*, when set loose at a buffet.

Americans consume more than 50 billion gallons of soft drinks per year. That's about a gallon per week per person. If all the Coca-Cola ever produced was put in eight-ounce bottles laid end to end, it would reach the moon and back about 1300 times. Soft drinks now are made with HFCS to save money in manufacturing.

The Center for Science in the Public Interest said research showed teenagers consume an average of two to three cans of soda per day in the United States. The percentage of overweight children in the United States has tripled since 1980. Public health advocacy group, the Center for Science in the Public Interest, said soda was "liquid candy" and called for cigarette style health warnings on cans.

HFCS isn't the only culprit in soda however. Phosphoric Acid interferes with your body's ability to use calcium, which can lead to osteoporosis or softening of the teeth and bones. Phosphoric acid also neutralizes the hydrochloric acid in your stomach, which can interfere with digestion, making it difficult to utilize nutrients. Caffeine cause jitters, insomnia, high blood pressure, irregular heartbeat, elevated blood cholesterol levels, vitamin and mineral depletion, breast lumps, birth defects, and perhaps some forms of cancer. These are just a couple of the many ingredients in soda pop that can cause health issues, so stay away and keep your kids away from this effective poison!

HFCS isn't seen by the brain as sugar (or a food at all), so it doesn't turn off the hunger signals like other sugars. Diet food manufacturers know this and use it as an ingredient so you will eat more of their product! Sugar, and HFCS are simply the worst "food" ingredients available.

Hydrogenated fats and trans fats are also poisons to your body. This 3rd place winner is found in so many processed foods, it's amazing anyone is still alive! These fats are known to cause cancer and a host of other health problems, but we still eat them because they give junk food its appeal. They are also addicting, so the more we eat them, the more we crave them.

Junk food manufacturers know good and well that most of the ingredients in their products are completely unnecessary for any other purpose than to get you physically hooked. Most of us agree that natural potato chips *taste* the best, but we *crave* the junk chips because of the long ingredient list filled with addictive chemicals.

It really is a conspiracy, and the food industry knows it, but it's all about profit (at your expense), and that's OK by them! They know they are sending you to the hospital and eventually to an early grave, but as long as they get paid, they can laugh all the way to the bank. Ninety percent of the money spent on groceries last year went towards the purchase of processed foods. One hundred years ago, it was exactly opposite, with ninety percent spent on real food like unprocessed meat and vegetables, and only ten percent spent on processed foods.

Hydrogenated and trans fats cause many diseases and health complications as well. We need healthy fats to stay alive but we don't need any of them in the form of hydrogenated or trans fats. These types of fats only lead to ill health and exaggerated fat storing properties.

Notice that "fat" wasn't listed first in this section. That's because we need to eat some healthy fat to lose fat. If you cut all fats out of your diet, you would suffer health complications and would have a very hard time getting lean. When people go on a "fat free" diet, they often lose weight in the beginning, but quickly plateau when their body realizes it isn't getting enough of this important macronutrient. It switches into survival mode and holds on to the fat it has, in order to preserve its health in case it is in some kind of a "fat famine."

Some fat is vital to a healthy body. Fat covers your nerves and protects your organs, so the body recognizes the importance of this tissue. Your body also sees it as a valuable energy reserve. Women need more fat on their bodies than men, but everyone is different.

Some women shouldn't get below 20 percent body fat, while others can go down to single digits and stay healthy. Men can usually go under 10 percent body fat with little or no problem, but everyone will find it harder to lose fat the leaner they get because of the body's natural tendency to preserve a minimum amount for proper health and survival.

Certain carb and fat combinations take the award for the fourth worst metabolism reducer. Sugar and fat together is a great way to slow your fat burning metabolism and increase your fat storage mode. Things like cookies, chips, white bread and butter, and even baked potatoes and gravy will make your fat cells swell the fastest.

Choosing your types and amounts of carbs and fat combinations carefully—especially in the evening-will go a long way toward stopping the fat gain. The wrong kinds of carbs and combinations with fat will also turn you into a fat storing machine. Fat will do very little to increase your metabolism because the body doesn't have to do any work to store it, since it is already converted.

Carbs can augment this storage process because they typically increase insulin levels which cause the storage mechanisms to turn on. This can be a good thing if it's protein you're trying to store in your muscles, but it can be a bad thing if you don't want to store fat.

Different kinds of carbs have different effects on insulin levels, so not all carbs will put your body in the storing mode. High glycemic carbs like flour, starches and sugars are the best at raising insulin levels and the low glycemic carbs like vegetables (especially dark greens) don't have this insulin elevation response. Not all carbs are bad and not all high glycemic carbs are bad either. It's just how you eat them, when, and with what that matters.

Refined flour takes fifth place because it is in so many foods, and the things they do to it in the refinement process would make your toes curl! Nutrients are lost almost completely, and the resulting substance is pure empty calories. Refined flour contributes absolutely zero to your health and only takes away from it due to increased insulin levels and fat storing ability.

The sixth worse culprit that will slow your metabolism is artificial sweeteners. These chemicals found in most junk foods, sodas, sweets and "diet" or "low carb" items are straight poison to your fat burning factory. These toxins are not only physically addictive, but they also store in your fat cells making them harder to empty out and be burned off!

The food industry knows the addictive qualities of these toxins and adds more than necessary so you get hooked and keep buying their food! Even the "diet" food companies don't want you to lose weight because if you do, they don't get to sell you any more food. They spend their money marketing the illusion of weight loss so you keep buying it and failing over and over.

Certain ingredients found in diet foods are also designed to be "triggers" that increase your craving for sugar and fat. This causes you to give in and eat the foods you shouldn't so you stay fat. Then you blame yourself and not them, and you keep buying their diet foods, perpetuating the cycle.

These artificial sweeteners include high fructose corn syrup, Aspartame, Acesulfame potassium, Sucralose, Saccharin, Cyclamate, and Neotame. We have been brainwashed to believe that these chemicals will lower our calorie intake by substituting sugar to help us lose fat. This may work initially, but even if it does, this will level off quickly and then become a plateau that is very hard to break because of the newly created "stubborn" fat due to the chemical build up in the fat cells.

These artificial lab-created chemicals are all poison to your body, and especially your fat metabolism. Even Sucralose (Splenda brand) is far from natural as the makers claim. It is indeed derived from sugar, but the process of popping off sugar molecules and adding chlorine molecules makes it unhealthy for any living thing.

Pure unrefined sugar and organic honey are the only sweeteners that won't poison your system. The problem with both of them is they will still elevate your insulin and cause you to go into a fat storing mode. They will also compete with vitamin absorption at the cell membrane, which can weaken your immune system.

The only safe sweetener that has no negative effects on fat storage or immune function is Stevia. It is derived from the Stevia plant and undergoes no lab alterations or refinements. It also contributes no calories because the serving size is about 300 times smaller than sugar. Some even claim it aids digestion as a probiotic and helps to populate your intestines with healthy microbes. You can add it to anything and even cook with it so why not use it?

Stevia is a win-win for your fat cells and your health. Sometimes it is combined with inulin fiber and other times with lactose. These are harmless additions that are meant to aid in cooking and serving size simplifications, but if you can find it in pure form, that is the best way to go.

The seventh worse metabolism reducer is farmed and processed meats. I am definitely "pro-meat" but not the kind most of us eat. Non-organic chicken, beef, turkey, or almost anything else is full of chemicals, pesticides, drugs and hormones. Many people have been driven to becoming vegans after a little education into how the animals are raised and what the farmers are putting into them!

Non-organic animals are cooped up in cages or pens to prevent them from getting healthy exercise! This forced sedentary life makes the meat fatter and more tender so you think it takes better. These raising techniques combined with the toxic additives make for a fat storing mode that won't stop. Your body sees these harmful molecules and reduces storage of the beneficial protein as well.

The only way around it is to buy certified organic meat from free range farms. If the animals are walking around looking for their own clean food (instead of cooped up and fed pesticide laden grain, antibiotics and hormones) they will produce leaner natural meat. This meat is recognized by the body as an absorbable protein source and is then used and converted to muscle. This results in an increased metabolism instead of a decreased one.

SEVEN EASY WAYS TO STOKE YOUR METABOLISM DURING THE DAY

1.) Eat to your hunger scale. Rate your hunger from 1-10, and only eat when you are at a 6-7. Then stop when you are at a 3-4. Keeping this small hunger window will make sure your metabolism is always occupied with food and won't shut down into survival mode. It will also ensure you don't overeat which can create an insulin spike that puts you in a fat storing mode.

2.) Take stairs up and elevators down. No more escalators or elevators to get you to higher floors! Traveling the vertical component with your body burns about 10 times more energy than walking flat, and about 100 times more energy than standing still (as on an elevator).

If you doubt this, try it yourself. Compare how you feel after walking 1,000 steps around town to how you feel after walking 1,000 stairs up a building (or 50 floors). It will take you only about 100 stairs (or 5 floors) however, to see what I mean. Avoid going back down stairs though, because the impact on your joints is more detrimental than the benefit of the exercise involved.

I recently competed in a local stair climb competition up a skyscraper in Seattle. I only trained for 7 weeks, and my workouts consisted of running up 63 floors 2-4 times a week in another Seattle skyscraper. The workout itself only took me 8 minutes, but the fat I lost was amazing. I actually had to eat carbs 4-5 times a week just to keep my fat up to 5-7% body fat so I didn't get too lean! How's that for a problem to have?

3.) Short intense exercise. When you are growing up, your metabolism is higher because your body is making new cells, growing bone, increasing muscle, producing hormones, etc. When you perform short, high intensity exercise sessions, your body is doing much of the same thing. It really is making you younger!

4.) Park your car in the farthest spot from the entrance at work and at the store. That nominal increase in walking distance each day won't be the physical answer to burning off fat, but you should do it for mental reasons. Every extra step you take is another confirmation that you are making a commitment to getting leaner each day. This affirmation will remind your subconscious to make this happen.

5.) Never sit still for more than one hour. This is more of a challenge for those of us who are at computers or on the phone all day long, but just getting up for a quick walk down the hall or up and down a flight of stairs can keep your metabolism from going to sleep from hours of sitting.

Even if you are trapped on a headset and a phone, you can still stand up and sit back down a few times instead of just sitting there dormant. The longer you sit in one place, the further your metabolism slips and the more your back vertebrae are stressed. Sitting is the most damaging posture you can have as far as your back is concerned, and worn out vertebrae make exercise harder and more painful, often starting a destructive downward spiral.

6.) Limit your TV viewing, but if you must watch it, do something at the same time. Stretch, do some crunches, pushups, or cook your food for the next day while watching your favorite show. I often use that time to do my rotator cuff exercises or clean the room to keep myself active while catching up on my shows.

7.) Activate your TEF. The thermic effect of food (TEF) is the amount of energy required for digestion and absorption of the food you eat. Digestion starts with chewing because this breaks food down for the stomach to digest easier. Chewing burns calories because your jaw muscles are "working out."

The longer you chew, the better this workout is, and you will burn more calories before you even swallow. This also keeps the food in your mouth longer, which gives your salivary glands time to do their job of breaking down nutrients properly.

This breakdown in your mouth is very important because you will actually store less fat and absorb more protein eating this way. Fat doesn't even need to be broken down, so if this is swallowed quickly without processing in the mouth, the body can still extract it and store it. For this reason fat contributes little to no TEF expenditure.

Protein in the other hand, is harder to process so if it is swallowed quickly without the aided oral breakdown, the stomach passes a larger percentage through without absorbing it. If you chew thoroughly, protein can contribute more than 10 times the TEF expenditure of fat! If swallowed quickly however, the TEF effect of protein can be cut in half.

Carbs are a different story. High fructose corn syrup has about the same TEF as fat. Simple carbs (especially refined sugars) contribute only about two times the TEF of fat. Starches bump it up to three times the TEF of fat, but complex carbs produce about four times fat TEF. Fiber carbs contribute even more because fiber binds to fat molecules in your stomach and helps pull these through preventing their absorption.

The TEF of protein is the main reason for always seeking out a high protein diet. This gives you a temporary metabolic elevation every time you eat. The other reason for a high protein diet is that you can build muscle easier which in turn raises your metabolism permanently due to the extra lean tissue on your frame.

Have emergency packs of high protein food sources with you during the day so when things get busy and you don't have time to eat, there is something available to keep your metabolism humming all day long.

CHAPTER THIRTEEN

CRACKING YOUR METABOLIC SET POINT CODE

Once you have turned the corner into a fat burner, it's not over. You need to maintain your habits long enough to convince your body to permanently adopt this new metabolism. Once it has, your new set point is achieved. As you continue to maintain your new set point, your genes will even change, and you can actually pass this on to your kids!

Studies now show that fat genes can be inherited from parents. Fat genes can have spontaneous beginnings as well. The crucial times for this phenomenon seem to be in the womb for girls and young adolescence for boys. If food habits are altered during these periods (i.e. overeating and junk foods), genes can actually change and pass the changes down to future generations.

The reverse is true as well however. Recent studies also show that you can alter your genes in the positive way just as well, and even turn yourself into a permanent fat burner. The longer you stay at your new set point once you reset it, the more time your genes have to change. Once these genes have changed, they are now a part of you and will also be a part of your future kids!

Resetting your set point takes longer for some and can be fairly quick for others. It depends largely on the genes you inherited, how long you have been at your previous set point, and your past history of fat loss and fat gain. Even the most messed up metabolisms, and the most stubborn set points can be fixed permanently, so there is hope for everyone!

Here is the news you probably haven't heard before (even if you are an expert in the field). Your metabolic set point is only half genetic, or more specifically, located in your cell's DNA. The other half of your set point is located in your brain! Both halves can be changed, so neither is permanent. Genes can be altered over time, and so can your brain's wiring.

The brain's metabolic set point is based on what you saw modeled growing up. This modeling came from your parents, TV, society, friends, teachers, and so on. You developed habits, cravings, and emotional eating patterns based on these past observations and personal experiences.

Even if people do lose weight on a diet, they usually rebound because of their brain's set point, not their genetic set point. The "experts" mistakenly attribute weight gain rebounds to the genetic set point, but that just doesn't make sense, because if someone can lose fat by following certain habits, they can certainly keep it off by sticking with those same habits. It's the brain's set point that causes the habits to relapse and the resulting fat to come back on.

People fall back into old eating patterns without even realizing it because of their mental wiring. This is why section one of this book is so important to read and re-read! You must rewire your brain and reset your metal set point if you wish to keep the fat off. Since keeping the fat off is the only way to alter your genetic set point, the horse must certainly come before the cart here!

The most important point to learn is that your thoughts are the key to changing your brain and your mental set point. Even if you don't believe yourself when you say, "I'm going to get leaner today," say it anyway, because it is a thought that your subconscious will buy into. Thoughts lead to feelings, feelings lead to actions, and actions lead to results.

Your subconscious controls your actions more than your conscious mind does, and programming your subconscious is as easy as repeating the messages you want it to believe, more than the messages you don't want it to believe. I know I'm repeating this point over and over, but that's part of the process isn't it? The most important thing you can do is to tell yourself every day (whether your conscious mind believes it or not) that you are getting leaner and that your metabolism is getting faster.

Thin people model that lifestyle, and can relate to other thin people. Fat people model that lifestyle, and relate to other fat people. Fat people are often resentful of thin people, and that attitude actually perpetuates the problem!

We are more likely to achieve a certain trait of we admire that trait. If you resent rich people, you are telling your brain over and over that is wrong or bad, and your subconscious will make darn sure that your actions prevent you from ever becoming rich. The same goes for your body. If you resent thin people, or find jealousy dominating your thoughts toward them, those thoughts will turn into negative feelings about thin people. These negative thoughts will cause your subconscious to change your actions and make you to stay fat.

If, instead, you force yourself to admire thin people, you will be more likely to become thin yourself. You can do this by sending a feeling of admiration to a thin person every time you see one. Think about blessing them instead of resenting them. Tell yourself every morning that you love thin people and are becoming one of them. Bless that which you want, and it will be yours. That which you negate, you will never have. It is really that simple!

While you are taking the first and most important step by changing your brain, you can also be working on changing your metabolism so you can get to your new set point as quickly as possible. As previously mentioned, muscle is your metabolism. Getting muscle takes the dedication and hard work, but maintaining it is actually less than half the work of getting it. This is good news because once you have the muscle, you must maintain it to keep your metabolism elevated and to reset your metabolism.

Resetting your metabolic rate takes different lengths of time for different people. Some can do it in a matter of weeks while others may take months or even a couple of years in some cases. Even in the most extreme cases, like individuals who came from a long line of obese ancestors, and have been overweight their whole lives can do it in two years or less. Two years might sound like a long time, but for someone who has been overweight for their whole life, this is a relatively short period of time and certainly worth it.

Once your metabolism is reset, you are much more resistant to holiday splurges and indiscretions, but be careful because you must continue to guard and protect it. Falling back on old habits and staying there can drag it back down over time to the place it used to be!

A normal healthy set point will typically not let your body fat change more than 10% in a short period. An interesting study showed this phenomenon clearly. A group of people were instructed to eat as much food as they could all day every day for 2 months. They were also told to remain as sedentary as possible. After an initial spike in fat gain, these people leveled off, and despite continued calorie intake well past their metabolic calculations, they just got hot and sweaty instead of fatter. Their metabolisms were simply choosing to burn off the extra food instead of converting it and storing more past their set points.

Most of us work this way. If we continue to hammer away at this set point limit however, it will give in and adjust up, allowing us to get fatter. The time it takes for that to happen differs between people based on genetics, history, muscle mass, and how long the set point was maintained.

SEVEN MOOD ELEVATORS FOR OPTIMAL FAT BURNING HORMONE RELEASE

It is a fact that happy people burn more fat. Fat people may seem more "jolly" but in most cases, that is an outward "mask" for a very unhappy person on the inside. True and consistent happiness releases the hormones and chemicals in your body to burn fat and increase your metabolism, so work on this every day!

1.) Go to your happy place. Synthetic happiness is the same as experience happiness as far as the brain is concerned. The brain does not know the difference between remembering a happy moment and actually experiencing that moment. The same positive chemical changes take place whether it is real or imagined.

Every positive thought you have causes a release of certain hormones for up to four hours that help you to burn fat and build muscle! The opposite is true of negative emotions however, so it is important to catch yourself thinking those thoughts and turn on your good mood.

2.) Shed some light on it. Seasonal affective disorder or SAD is quite common and goes largely unaddressed because most victims don't know they have it. This is caused by too little sunshine for too long, and is most common in northern latitudes. It can be remedied with light therapies—namely full spectrum lighting. These lights can be put in your existing lamps at home and can also be purchased as a stand alone system.

3.) Tune in a funny station. Find a comedy station next time you are driving or play a funny CD to make you laugh. Each laugh is a full dose of hormones that burn off your fat. The saying, "laughter is the best medicine" really is correct. We just didn't know how accurate and literal that was until science recently confirmed it.

4.) Practice contentment. This is a skill and with practice, will prove invaluable. It will help you focus on your positives and the areas that are changing for the better. Content people eat less often and in smaller amounts. There is no emotional void they are trying to fill, because they are happy about who they are and with what they have.

5.) Show appreciation. Tell someone you appreciate them and watch how that makes you both feel. Just thinking about being thankful for something will release fat burning chemicals through your body.

6.) Give a gift to someone for no reason. Just tell them it was simply because you were thinking of them. Seeing their day light up will actually light yours up even more, and will ignite your fat burning furnace.

7.) Tell someone you love them. I saved the best technique for last. The act of loving someone is the most powerful mood elevator of all, and has the longest positive hormone release of anything you can do. Even thinking about love towards someone will cause your levels to elevate.

CHAPTER FOURTEEN

CRACKING YOUR BODY TYPE CODE

There are three main body types, and your genetics predispose you toward one of them. Most people are a combination of a couple of different types, but there certainly are a few pure body types as well. The three types of physique are ectomorph, mesomorph, and endomorph. The ectomorphs are long, lean and wiry. Mesomorphs are more square shaped with muscular tendencies. Endomorphs are typically pear shaped and become overweight fairly easily.

Most ectomorphs are also called "hard gainers" because muscle comes slowly and requires more work to keep it on. They also lose muscle fast when not exercising. Although ectomorphs have a difficult time adding muscle, they usually gain fat slower as well. People either add tissue easily or they don't, and it's usually all types of tissue instead of specifically fat or muscle. Those who are genetically predisposed to add muscle easier like the mesomorphs also gain fat easier. Mesomorphs tend to hang on to muscle better than others, but the same goes for their fat tissue.

An easy test to find out if you are an ectomorph is to grab your own wrist around its largest part where the bony knob sticks out (if this knob isn't prominent skip this test because you're not an ectomorph). If you can touch your pinky finger to your thumb you're probably an ectomorph. Try both sides because they may be different. A positive test on one side is definitive, but if you can pass this test on both sides, you are almost certainly an ectomorph.

Ectomorphs don't usually have large appetites. They may be able to eat a high volume of food in one sitting but they can also go long periods of time without eating, and suffer few hunger pangs. At the end of the day their calories are typically low, and if they do spike for a day or two it is usually followed by a low calorie day with little to no hunger.

This low calorie intake isn't problematic by itself, because calories don't really matter as much as macronutrients, but it almost always causes a low protein intake to coincide. Low protein will hamper muscle growth. Low carbs will also hamper muscle growth because carbs are what helps the absorption of protein. If they are both low, as the case with most ectomorphs because of a natural decreased appetite, protein will have a hard time adding itself to the muscle for building purposes.

Ectomorphs have to commit to taking in about twice the protein of other body types. They need about one gram per pound of bodyweight as a daily minimum. They also need to spread that throughout the day so their muscles always have a ready supply to pull from the bloodstream. 20 grams every couple of waking hours is a good habit to get into for regular and optimal absorption. 40 grams within five minutes of a strength training or anaerobic workout is also vital, because this is the time the muscles are searching the hardest for protein. The second most important time for the best protein absorption is in the morning, so make sure you get some to start off your day.

Water is another key ingredient because muscles are 75 percent water. Ectomorphs need a constant supply of this as well to build muscle, so drinking consistently through the day will make this task easier to accomplish. If each day is started with water and protein and then continued with regular doses of both through the day, with special attention to post workout supply, muscle can be gained as easily as possible for the ectomorph.

Ectomorphs need extra help in absorbing protein so a low-carb kind of diet is not the best idea for muscle gain. Carbs should accompany protein for proper absorption. Remember that the insulin spike puts you in a storing mode for all macronutrients, so this will help it get to your muscles. Fat doesn't matter as much because it will usually take care of itself when you up your total intake of the other two macronutrients.

Training intensity is the final key to faster muscle gain. No matter what your body type, muscles have to fail to see the need for change. If they successfully perform whatever you're doing, they think they are fine "as-is" and will stay where they are. If they fail however, and can't do what is being asked of them, they will see the need to get stronger and improve. It really is this simple, so make sure your intensity is well beyond what you think is possible.

Even following all this advice to the "T" still may not produce results as fast as other body types, so you may have to just settle for a smaller frame and less muscle mass. Ectomorphs will never get on the cover of Muscle Mag, but they do often grace the covers of fitness magazines. You will have to be content with the chiseled, defined and "ripped" look over the bulky look.

The good news is that 99 percent of women and 94 percent of men surveyed prefer the fitness look over the bulky look anyway, so ectomorphs really have it made when it comes to the popular body image. Only a very small segment of the population thinks bodybuilders are physically attractive, so chalk that one up for the ectomorphs!

If you are not an ectomorph and still find it hard to gain muscle, you should still follow the advice above but with one exception: watch the simple carbs and fat intake because you will gain fat easier than ectomorphs. If you are in this group, you are probably and endomorph. This body type stores fat easily and loses it slowly. Resetting your metabolism as mentioned in the previous section will take the longest of any body type, but it is just as possible.

Endomorphs also have lower hormone levels that help to gain muscle, so this might be the most frustrating body type of all. Fat is hard to lose and muscle is hard to gain. It's not fair, but given enough time, endomorphs can look great as well. They tend to end up looking like competitive swimmers—long, toned and lean but not typically "ripped" with the muscle definition of the naturally lean ectomorphs.

Endomorphs also tend to be the body type most prone to obesity. This comes with other serious health risks as well. Recent scientific discoveries have found that obese men diagnosed with prostate cancer have more than 2 ½ times the risk of dying from the disease when compared to men of normal weight (March 2007 issue of *Cancer*). Obese men also have a 3 ½ times greater risk of cancer spreading to other organs than their thinner counterparts.

The link between obesity, prostate cancer and death is believed to involve hormones and inflammation. Obesity turns into an inflammatory disease as a by product and has negative affects on many functions and health aspects of the body ranging from circulation issues to terminal illness.

Two other studies found that obese men also experience a sharp decline in testosterone levels, while obese girls show much higher levels of the hormone than girls of normal weight. Testosterone is considered a male hormone, but it is found in females as well. Its functions include maintaining muscle mass, bone density, sex drive and energy levels, to name a few.

Testosterone levels naturally decline as men age, but scientists found that those who put on as little as 30 pounds of excess weight lost as much testosterone as if they had aged 10 years (Journal of Clinical Endocrinology and Metabolism, December 2006).

In a separate study in the same issue, researchers found that obese girls had 2-9 times the amount of testosterone than girls of normal weight. Many undesirable side effects of excess testosterone in girls range from excess hair growth to increased risk of diabetes.

Yet another study found that obese couples have a more difficult time conceiving than couples of normal weight. Researchers published in the March 2007 issue of Human Reproduction found that obese couple's chances of having to wait longer than a year before a woman conceived were nearly 3 times higher than couples of normal weight.

Only 30 percent of adults consider themselves overweight. The US government however, estimates that more than 60 percent of adults are overweight or obese. Of those who were overweight, only about 30% were worried about disease as a result.

A 2007 report from Trust for Americas Health cited that obesity rates rose in 31 states in 2006. Twenty-two states reported an increase for the second year in a row, and no states decreased. Obesity is now an official epidemic, and it's not just the endomorphs that share in this statistic. All body types can end up obese.

The mesomorph is the body type who gains all tissue easily. Muscle and fat both come fast, and strength is quickly acquired without much effort. Losing fat is a challenge however, so it is a trade off. World-class bodybuilders are always this body type. Mesomorphs lose muscle slowly when not exercising and seem to hold onto strength much longer once they have received it. The same goes for fat tissue however, so they have to take the good with the bad.

Mesomorphs tend to be the most athletic as well, and respond quickly to exercise. Their workouts burn more fat than other body types and protein is more easily absorbed without such a high need for carbs as with ectomorphs. Water is the most important component for the mesomorph, as they dehydrate quickly and sweat more than others during training.

Mesomorphs have to watch what they eat more closely to lose the fat, and maintain their workouts during strict nutrition to keep from losing muscle at the same time. This extra effort can be seen among any competitive bodybuilder as evidenced in their mood when getting close to a contest!

Endomorphs are the body type which really gets the shaft. They do gain muscle faster than the ectomorphs, but not as fast as the mesomorphs. They do however, pack on fat faster than any body type and have the hardest time losing it as well. Their bones are medium size, and their fat to muscle ratio is pretty poor by any standards.

Endomorphs are characteristically soft and have the most weight stored around their middle. Their metabolisms are usually slow and so is their physical pace. It takes more effort to lose fat than a mesomorph, and endomorphs find gaining muscle to be almost as hard as an ectomorph.

It certainly isn't fair to be born an endomorph, but the good news is there is the same hope for fitness and a lean body style as any other body type. It just takes more work. Once and endomorph resets his or her metabolic set point however, they can maintain it well and even pass down a more favorable body type to their kids.

No matter what your type, it will always seem to you that muscle comes on slow and fat comes on fast. You will also notice that muscle is lost rapidly and fat at a much slower pace. This is the way all of us are built, so we just have to learn to deal with it and work on contentment and patience to achieve our goals in the end and keep them for life.

Muscle comes slowly because it has to be built. This building process takes a long time and has to go through many different steps with lots of factors all lining up perfectly. Fat stores easily because it just has to be stored. Building is much more difficult than storing.

Muscle is a very high maintenance tissue so it leaves the body quickly as well. Your body will always try to burn the least amount of energy possible, and since muscle uses so much energy, the body will constantly try to rid itself of this tissue to increase its own efficiency. "Use it or lose it" certainly rings true for muscle tissue.

Fat is a no-maintenance tissue but provides maximum energy potential, so the body will store this up easily and put it in areas around the center of your mass (waist, butt and hips) to make it easier to haul around. This is why we have to work at gaining muscle, but not working at all gains fat.

All body types will lose muscle when they stop working out. Muscle is lost at different rates for different types, but everyone seems to panic when they know they will be on a vacation or away for a while with no access to exercise. Don't worry, because even if you can't exercise for a while (i.e. injury, new colicky baby, etc.), you won't be "starting from scratch" like you might fear.

It only takes as long as your break was (or sooner) to get back to where you were. If an ectomorph has worked out for a year and takes a month off, they aren't starting over. They will only take a month to regain the fitness they had. Mesomorphs can get fitness back even faster than their break, and endomorphs fall somewhere in the middle.

You will never be able to pick up your fitness program right where you left off, but you will notice your progress is much more accelerated because your muscles remember where they were and get back there much faster. You already laid down the protein and did the hard work in the past. Now it's just a matter of relaying the same protein in the same places.

Creating muscle initially takes more work because you have to effectively dig out pockets in the muscle cell for the protein to fill up. When you take a break, the protein gets taken out of the pockets fast, but the pockets themselves stay there. Then it is just a matter of sticking the protein back into those same pockets. No new "digging" has to take place.

Remember that different body types also measure and weigh differently. Ignore your scale weight and go with how your clothes are fitting to gauge your results. The Body Mass Index (BMI) is also a relatively worthless tool. Circumference measurements will also vary greatly based on different frames even if body fat measurements are the same between people. Never compare yourself to others. We are all different, and we all have our own relative level of fitness. If you compete only with yourself, and celebrate your own fitness improvements relative to your own specific goals, you will achieve true fitness and contentment.

CHAPTER FIFTEEN

CRACKING YOUR STRENGTH CODE

Strength training is the single most important factor in permanently raising your metabolism. Muscle is your metabolism, so the more you have, the higher your metabolic rate will be. This doesn't mean you have to bulk up. In fact, the unique protocols in this book will limit your capabilities for that. It simply means your muscle must change right down to the cellular level so it becomes an active fat furnace instead of a sedentary inactive tissue.

I only weigh 170 lbs, but have the metabolism of a much heavier person. This is due to the way my muscles have formed and how they operate. I can temporarily raise my metabolism through the type and timing of my food, but my metabolism is also running full steam ahead while I am asleep because of the kind of lean tissue I have developed.

The muscle you will acquire through the protocols in this book will be denser than you would get with traditional training. Since you will be training both strength and endurance, the muscle cell grows in size much more slowly, but changes internally very fast.

Traditional strength training will cause you to bulk up. This is why most women don't like it. Traditional methods were invented for this purpose and still work pretty well for that goal. They take a lot of time, but the multiple sets and reps with very little time under load cause this response. Since the muscle is only training for 10-15 seconds during a set and then gets a rest, oxygen is not needed.

The capillaries that carry the oxygen are on the outside of the muscle, and the mechanisms that use that oxygen for energy are located in the nucleus which is deeper in the muscle, located in the muscle fibers themselves. If oxygen is not needed, the muscle allows itself to bet bigger and increases the space between the capillaries and the nucleus.

If the set is longer than 30 seconds, the oxygen system is needed, so the muscle will shrink in circumference to get the capillaries closer to the nucleus and increase the efficiency of this energy system. Marathon runners may look like they have less muscle than a bodybuilder but they don't. Their cells are just shrunk down to increase their aerobic energy system efficiency.

The fast motion and ballistic nature of traditional training also encourage the muscle to increase in girth so it is more resistant to injury, because it recognizes that this style has a high potential for injury. A thicker cell is harder to tear, just like a string or rope. The methods in this book, however, will not significantly increase the circumference of the cell, but with the density increase will make it more resistant to injury, much like a thin cable is stronger than a thick rope.

The fitter and stronger I get, the less I have to work out. This is a reverse of traditional training which requires more time to support bigger muscles like a competitive bodybuilder. These poor saps end up training 8-12 hours a day for continued improvement!

I have reached contentment with my body, so I am happy with where I am. I now strength train just 20 minutes, once a week for maintenance. I trained 20 minutes twice a week to get where I am, but now need to train only half that amount of time. I used to train 2 hours a day, 6 days a week for very slow results that eventually stagnated in a long and nasty plateau.

This lack of progress for a massive time investment was a frustration to say the least, and was what started me on my research quest to find a better way. Cutting the time down and increasing the intensity was a gamble to me, but I was willing to try anything.

I actually didn't think my initial experiments would work, but the more I tried them, the better shape I got into and my strength went through the roof. I continued to get stronger and more toned each year, and the rest is history. I am still developing new methods and will continue to refine the system until new research stops coming out, which I can't see ever happening, so my methods will only continue to improve.

A complete bibliography is included on the website *www. crackingyourcode.com* because including all the studies in this book would have made it too long. The science I cite in this book is also based on more than one study or group of scientists, so even listing names would add too much length to the book. If I were to include all the studies I have used to develop these methods, the book would have been another 90 pages longer and that's a lot of trees!

At my personal training centers (the X Gyms), we call our techniques the "Triple Sevens" methods. We have 7 methods we use on our clients; most exercise routines include 7 exercises, and the routines and protocols are changed every 7 weeks. Because most of these protocols are too complicated to explain with words, I have simplified the program in this book to three methods, and have modified them so you can get maximum benefit with little to no help from anyone else.

The science behind the methods is important to understand because most other traditional methods were created without any science at all. They were just some person's idea that seemed to work for them personally and then became a "fad" that grew into a movement. The following points spell out the differences with the methods in this book and explain the additional benefits you will enjoy.

1. Triple Sevens (TS) prevents adaptation. Each program lasts 7 weeks (usually the soonest someone can adapt to a routine), and is then changed. The change need only be minor to cause the muscles and systems to begin a new and fresh improvement curve. This regular technique change, along with exercise switches, will ensure that the different metabolic and skeletal muscular systems are all trained evenly and thoroughly.
2. TS helps prevent athletic injuries. Through the different protocols, tissues strengthen evenly, and tendon growth is promoted at the same rate as the muscle. Since conventional training causes the tendon strength increases to lag behind the muscle, those methods cause a much stronger muscle to pull on a slightly stronger tendon, making it more likely to "pop"-especially among recreational athletes like weekend basketball, soccer, football, or tennis players, etc.
3. For bone density to increase, there are three main contributing factors: amount of force applied, rate of speed, and direction of force. Bone density is only minimally increased with conventional training because of the uncontrolled nature and motion in only one plane. TS has different routines and specific techniques addressing these factors, maximizing bone density improvement. It begins

with small, controlled movements with light weights to strengthen the musculature, but then moves on to other methods and splinter techniques that utilize this new muscle power to specifically maximize bone density.

4. TS gives you aerobic conditioning while it is strengthening you at the same time. The more fit you are aerobically, the more mitochondria you have in your muscles. This raises your metabolism, making you burn more calories during exercise *and* rest. You will also recover faster between sets and between workouts if you enjoy a more efficient and trained aerobic system.

   Still further, it should be noted that too much aerobic conditioning can slow optimum muscle growth and strength improvement. This is why I recommend anaerobic interval training. If your emphasis *is* on endurance competitions, TS would still assist in improvement of your times, performance and strength, but you would have to do long duration exercise which will likely reduce your strength improvement rates.

5. TS recognizes individual differences and realizes that people all adapt at different rates and have different body types, fiber types, preferences, and mechanical differences necessitating different programs. This is why TS has multiple protocols and splinter techniques. The myofibrils, which contribute 20-30% of the muscle cell's makeup are best trained using a low rep set. The mitochondria which make up 15-25% of a cell, are best trained with longer duration contractions. The sarcoplasm, which makes up another 20-30% of the cell is best trained with medium duration contractions. TS hits all of these with specific variation between protocols changing every 7 weeks, ensuring well-rounded fitness of all the systems.

This multi-protocol concept is unique to this system. Other books and exercise systems will have you change exercises and even emphasis, periodically, from strength training to endurance training, but the rep itself goes unchanged. Plateaus are unavoidable because the muscle will adapt to that particular type of rep and contraction speed.

When you use these methods, the very nature of the basic rep changes along with the exercises. This will truly prevent plateaus and give your muscle a well-rounded fitness that applies to the real world and lots of different practical situations.

What to Expect From This Strength Training System

In your first 7 weeks, you will be doing the "Ratchets" protocol. This method targets a specific energy system and muscle fiber type. It will develop strength as well as coordination. During this first phase your muscles will improve their "innervation," meaning the nerves telling your muscles to contract are becoming healthier and more efficient. This makes you stronger without a significant increase in muscle fiber size.

During this phase women may begin to feel more toned and tight, and men may notice some improvement in muscle definition, shape and form. Muscle innervation must happen first before hypertrophy (fiber size increase) can begin. The hypertrophy stage won't start until the innervation phase has run its course, which usually takes about 5-7 weeks.

You will fall somewhere within a bell-shaped curve for improvement rates. A few will be all the way to the right side of the curve and may see visible results after their first four sessions! The other minority on the opposite side of the curve may have to wait two months or more before seeing obvious changes in the mirror.

If you're in this "slow changers" group, you'll become impatient around the 4th or 5th week, and pretty frustrated that no visible results are happening. This is quite understandable because you've been working hard and would like a return for your efforts, but just hang in there and wait your body out. It will give in eventually and when it does, it all pays off. You can also move yourself out of that group over time by improving your metabolism as your muscle tissue changes.

The majority fall within the middle portion of the curve and begin to see changes within the first protocol (7 weeks), and even more marked results during their second protocol. Progress is constant, and within about 8 months, goals are often achieved. Regardless of which group you are in, the results you will experience will be at least double those of conventional training.

Results differ from person to person, so don't compare yourself to someone else. You may have a friend who is at the right side of the bell curve. You however, may be on the left side of the bell curve. It is all based on your hormone levels, protein uptake ability, genetics, body composition, resistance to change, and personal and family history, to name just a few variables.

It's the little things you will notice first, like the groceries feel lighter when you pick them up, or walking up the stairs is easier than before. Enjoy this progress and focus on these small changes. They can be expected during your first 7 weeks as muscle innervation runs its course. Next, you will notice that your muscles feel tighter and things "jiggle" less. You may even begin to see some size changes if you are a man.

Your next protocol will be the "Mid Stops" method and your final protocol will be the "Tiered" method. This method change every 7 weeks will also be accompanied by a change in exercises. Changing both of these components every 7 weeks will keep your muscles in the innervation phase and out of the muscle bulking phase. You will see strength gain and muscle tone gains beyond what you have experienced in the past, but without the usual increase in girth.

Another benefit you will see from this program is in your motor skill development. You will notice sports become easier as your coordination improves. Your pain tolerance will also increase, allowing you to endure longer with physical tasks and sports you previously found too unpleasant.

Consistency is the key to progress with this system. You must stick to the *twice a week* regimen for proper consistency. If you miss a workout, make it up at a different time. The twice a week frequency was created on purpose, based on the latest research, and is vital to your rate of progress.

Optimum nutrition allows your muscles to recover and gives them the tools to rebuild. They will change only as fast as you allow them to, by supplying them with the proper nutrients. Muscles are 75% water and 25% protein. This is why I emphasize both so much. Please be sure to heed the nutritional advice in this book for optimal strength improvement and metabolic elevation.

Cardiovascular exercise makes the initial weight loss easier by burning more fat and temporarily raising your metabolism. It also improves your recovery rate between sessions, making your muscles more ready for the next strength workout, and maximizing the benefit from the previous one. Be sure to carefully follow the cardio section in this book as well, for maximal strength improvements.

Consistency with the strength workouts, proper nutrition, and regular cardio will all work together to give you the results you are after. *The 20 minute workout by itself is not a quick weight loss program.* It is a permanent fat loss program *over time* because your metabolism will be increasing and habits will change, but short-term reduction also depends on the other factors. How closely you follow the formulas here will dictate how rapidly your results are realized.

In the beginning you will experience a few new sensations. These protocols cause an endorphin high unlike other exercise programs. The high intensity nature also reduces stress levels drastically. This training style has been proven through recent research to be the most effective form of exercise for stress reduction, so you are on your way to busting your stress by acting on the principles in this book!

Stress and emotions are stored in our muscles and soft tissue. High intensity exercise effectively "squeezes" them out through the maximal muscle contraction process. I just trained one of my trainers yesterday who hadn't worked out for a couple of weeks due to factors and stressful situations in her life beyond her control. She almost cried several times during the workout because so many emotions were being released. Afterward, she felt as if a giant weight had been lifted that she didn't even know was there! Her endorphins were elevated as well, and the combination of these effects made her feel as if she had just received months of therapy in a psychologist's office.

This stress reduction and endorphin release can make you quite excited about the program, and with the newfound strength, the "honeymoon" phase begins. If you follow the nutritional prescriptions included in the program you will also see muscular changes about the time the 'honeymoon" period starts to wear off, so this will keep you going with renewed enthusiasm that often becomes addicting.

This is a fitness *system*, not just a bunch of workouts like outdated conventional strength training. There is a big difference. These workouts by themselves are vastly superior to conventional workouts, but are also a part of an overall *system* including cardio and nutrition advice pulling from research as recent as *the year this book was published*!

Let's get right to the nitty gritty. The exercises pictured in this first section can be done in your home with no equipment needed. This is a great starting routine as well if you are new to strength training. Proper form is crucial, so make sure you are following the pictures as best you can. Use a mirror to check your form because feeling a movement and seeing it can be quite a different experience.

The exercises and techniques in this book are the safest available. Any exercise however, comes with risks, so make sure you are first cleared by your doctor to do high intensity exercise, and listen to your body during your workouts. Don't assume you aren't suited for high intensity training either. Some people use advanced age, injuries, physical limitations, or poor condition as an excuse, so let your doctor decide if it is right for you.

If you feel joint pain or "bad pain" anywhere in the muscles, tendons or other tissue, stop immediately and make an appointment to get it checked out with a medical professional before continuing that movement. Remember that for every exercise you do, there are 101 alternative exercises for that same muscle that might be OK with a different angle or technique.

Pushing through the muscle "burn" is what needs to happen for the muscle to change and improve. Pushing through bad pain or joint pain will only cause you to go backward or stagnate in your progress. You will quickly learn the difference between these types of pain, but pay special attention to your joints, lower back, and neck.

A new strength workout might take up to 30 minutes to complete, but as you learn it and build skill within the protocol, it will only take 15-20 minutes with proper execution. Each protocol is different and some take longer than others, but even the most time consuming protocol will still fall within the 20 minute limit.

Remember that failure is the key. This is the most important aspect to your training program, and must be the goal for the workout to provide the benefits intended. If your muscle can do it, it won't see a need to change because it thinks it is fine "as is." If it can't do it, it sees the need to change, and if provided the right nutrients as building blocks, will rebuild stronger, firmer, and more toned than before.

Muscles won't change if they don't have to. The human body was designed to be as efficient as possible. It only maintains a minimum amount of muscle because it is a high maintenance active tissue. If you sit all day, your body doesn't need as much, so it gets rid of it through atrophy, and if your calories exceed your sedentary burn rate, you will only gain fat as your bodyweight increases.

If muscles are kept active however, positive changes take place as they improve and grow to accommodate the activity. Extra calories can turn into muscle tissue instead of fat, and your metabolism will speed up instead of slow down.

Resistance training is in a class of its own with respect to lean tissue and metabolism improvement. It has been shown over the centuries to be the best way to improve both of these areas. The sad part is that most people don't understand how, and end up just spinning their wheels in a fruitless effort, simply wasting time as they try. The secret is muscle fatigue. As stated above, muscles will only change if they have to. The best way to make a muscle realize it has to change is to make it fail. Pushing to the point of physical failure forces adaptations and changes within the muscle, preparing it for success the next time. It realizes that it can't do what was just asked of it and therefore sees a reason to improve.

If fatigue isn't achieved, the muscle has no reason to change. It was successful. It says, "I can tolerate this, so I'm adequate as-is." This is how most people train. They push until it starts to burn and then quit. Even if they do multiple sets, they still end up merely spinning their wheels, never making any real progress.

I've seen people train for years and never change a bit. They might be getting some negligible temporary calorie expenditure during their session, but that quickly goes away and there is no long-term metabolism increase enjoyed.

On the other hand, I've seen people visibly change within just *four sessions* of high intensity X Gym training! Most take longer, but everyone enjoys results far surpassing any type of sub-fatigue training.

Muscle fatigue—to the point of failure and then beyond, is the necessary component for maximum gains in minimum time. The protocols I have developed are just ways to get to that magic point safer and faster, while cycling through different energy systems and fiber types for a well-rounded fitness and strength in the end.

Unloading the muscle or "offloading" as we call it at the X Gym, is when a client drops the weight or gives up momentarily due to mental failure. They get to the point of a burn or fatigue where they don't want to go on, or start to doubt if they can. This is most common among perfectionists and overachievers who don't want to experience muscle failure, or those who simply haven't yet developed the tolerance for full fatigue training.

The last rep—the one 3 or 4 past what you thought possible, is the one that brings the biggest results. All the reps leading up to it are just "rehearsal reps" or "prep reps" getting you ready for the "benefit rep" which is the one you fail at. Failure is good. It is showing the muscle it can't do it. When the muscle can't do something, it has to change. This is why the failure rep is so significant.

If you can complete the range, you're not done. Getting "stuck" is actually the goal, not a certain number of successfully completed reps. The difference between rapid change and stagnation lies solely in that one last rep that can't be completed successfully.

This system will take you further yet with splinter techniques to go **beyond** fatigue. This augments results even more, by creating an emergency situation inside the muscle, shocking it into drastic changes. This is why "hanging in there" will get you the results you never thought possible.

The strength training method itself is quite simple. There are only three protocols to learn, and two splinter techniques to master. Cycling through a new protocol every seven weeks will keep you from plateaus and from adapting to a particular routine.

This multi-protocol concept is one of the many unique ways this program is different from all the others. Traditional training will mix up the exercises every so often, but the reps themselves stay the same after a routine change, and the sets last roughly the same amount of time.

This lack of variety in how the rep is performed in traditional training creates the plateaus so many get frustrated with. The body adapts and can't figure out new ways to improve. We are created this way, so adaptation is normal. This is great for a distance runner, because as they adapt, they become more efficient.

For gaining strength and continued tone however, adaptation is a bad thing. Varying the exercises *and the method* prevents the adaptation from happening. The muscles can't get used to a particular movement pattern, so they have to keep changing and improving.

Changing methods also improves coordination as the nerves are trained harder with the motion variety. Traditional strength training is very fast, ballistic and uncontrolled, so the nerves actually become detrained and coordination gets worse.

If you have ever seen a professional bodybuilder try a sport they aren't familiar with, you have seen my point firsthand. They have detrained their coordination 8-12 hours every day in the gym, and their natural athletic ability goes out the window.

The frequency of your strength training sessions is important for optimal results as well. As long as you go to full fatigue within the method and then past fatigue with the splinters, you will only need to do one set per exercise and work out only twice a week.

Conventional training does indeed require 3 one hour sessions per week to see results. Muscles are broken down in such a way that 48 hours of recovery and rebuilding are required before the next exercise session. Years of experience have shown this to be true, and studies have recently confirmed it.

The methods in this book on the other hand, dictate different recovery patterns. The intensity is higher, and subsequent recovery takes longer. The muscles are actually broken down more than conventional training but with no cell damage, and the energy systems are taxed more deeply requiring longer rest between bouts.

Because of the speed of conventional training, microtears in the muscle fibers are commonplace, and scar tissue builds within the fibers. These torn fibers never heal and a resulting reduced force output is the end result. This scar tissue is partly responsible for the enormous size of bodybuilders' muscles. Since Triple Sevens protocols don't employ the fast ballistic movements and heavy weights of conventional training, microtears and scar tissue aren't a part of the growth and development process.

This leaves more intact fibers working to lift and pull, but a smaller girth and cross-sectional area. The strength-to-girth ratio of X Gym trained muscles compared to conventionally trained muscles is astounding. This is why X Gym clients develop a strength-to-weight ratio combined with high muscular endurance that only elite *athletes* possess.

Because energy systems are taxed along with muscle fibers, 2 days of rest is preferred between sessions. Those who have tried this system 3 times a week simply overtrain. The recovery window is too short and improvement is slowed (or even *declines* in some cases).

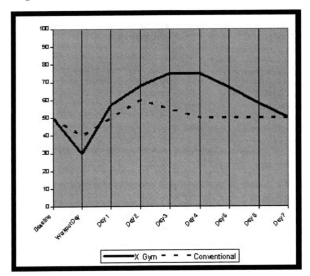

More than 4 days in between workouts on the other hand, can be too long. Muscles are great at atrophying. They do it well and rapidly because the body is trying to become more efficient through reducing this high maintenance tissue. The body will start undoing the results from a workout after about 4 days for this style of training or after 2 days for conventional training (see chart). After 7 days, almost all of the benefit from the workout is negated (or 4 with conventional training) and muscles return to baseline.

It is true that people have made improvements on one day a week with these methods. This is also amazing since the conventional school insists this is impossible. This improvement however, is slow and near flat line.

These methods also train the nerves as much as the muscles, so coordination is improved. I can take up a new sport now with more than twice the proficiency as when I was a teenager, because of this nerve training effect.

The first protocol in this multi-protocol concept is called ratchets. It involves creating 7 stops in the range of motion on the lifting phase and 7 stops on the lowering phase.

These stops needn't be too long. They just need to be long enough to be complete stops. If there is motion or bouncing, you aren't stopped. You will get better at the stops with time and as you do, it will take less time to come to a full stop. This is because your nerves are becoming trained, as mentioned before.

You will be doing 4-7 reps for each exercise. Count at the top of the rep so you know you have accomplished the hardest part of the range. Breathe when you feel like it. Timing your breaths doesn't matter. Everyone is different, so breathe when your body feels like it, and choose your frequency based on what feels natural to you. Just make sure you aren't holding your breath at any point. Constant airflow at all times is completely necessary.

It is also important to keep constant tension on the muscles and off of the joints. You will do this by keeping within the tension range instead of locking the joints at extension or resting at any point in the range.

This constant tension and no rest technique creates endurance and strength benefits at the same time. It also keeps your set shorter because fatigue is achieved faster. Since fatigue is the goal and not a certain number of reps, getting there in as little time as possible is paramount. Resting or taking breaks will only make you drag the set out longer, prolong your misery, and lengthen your workouts.

Full fatigue is the key to effective strength training. You should push to the point of complete muscle failure. You will know you are there because you "hit the wall" and can't continue moving. You are effectively "stuck" in position. This can happen at any point in the range, but usually occurs in the first half of the range.

When you reach the "wall", continue to hold that position for as long as you can. This will be 5-10 seconds. Once you can't hold it there any longer, start pulsing by moving just an inch up and down until you can't even do that any more and you start to sink down as gravity takes over.

These extra techniques to finish you off and ensure that fatigue has really happened are called "splinters" and must be accomplished to ensure full physical fatigue. If you achieve full fatigue and true physical failure, only one set is necessary. Research proves that even 3-5 additional sets beyond the initial full fatigue set gives no additional benefits.

This is great news for time-crunched people because each exercise will now take only 1-3 minutes! Doing one 2 minute set instead of 3-5 ten second sets with 2 minute rests in between is a huge time saver over traditional training, with much better results.

This type of training will strengthen you faster than traditional training because of the muscle failure. It will also build your endurance because of the long duration of the exercises. Traditional training actually detrains your endurance while strengthening your muscles at a slower rate.

The strength and endurance components combined together also prevent you from "bulking up" and increasing circumference measurements. Instead, you become long and lean with improved definition and tone to go along with your new strength. You will also become mentally stronger due to the fact you are pushing yourself to new limits.

The more you do this training, the better you will get at it, physically and mentally, with benefits to enjoy in both aspects. This is most apparent with my clients who ski. They tell me that they not only make it down the hill farther before they start to burn, but they also tell me they know they can now keep going through the burn!

THE RATCHET METHOD

Before you start the exercises in this or any routine, a warm up is necessary. This can be done by going for a 5 minute jog, climbing on a cardio machine, or just jumping up and down. Do whatever it takes to get your body warm. If your muscles are warm before you start strength training, they will be much stronger. Since you only get out of your workout what you put into it, more strength will certainly help your progress. The warm up will also make you less likely to be injured, so make sure this step always happens first.

Avoid stretching before you strength train. Research shows that this does nothing to warm you up or prevent injuries. In fact, it may make you more likely to be injured and will actually make you weaker. This will, of course, work against you in your strength workout, so stick to the warm up only before you train.

Each exercise requires only 4-7 reps in perfect form. If you can do 7, you are ready to move up in weight or the next form level. If you can't do 4, it's too heavy, and you should move down in weight or to change form. Always judge form very strictly. If you cheat your way to 7 reps, you will be progressing faster than your muscles are ready to, and you will overweight yourself, causing stagnation in strength. Struggling along with a weight that is too heavy is a sure way to flat line your progress and cheat yourself of optimal results.

If you can do 7 reps, go straight into your holds and pulses just as if you had reached failure. You will have to hold and pulse longer to get to full fatigue than if you had reached fatigue within the reps, but that's all part of the program. Remember that you are getting strength and endurance with these methods, so whether you fatigue quickly or not, you will be spending a lot of time under tension and will be training your nerves just as much as your muscles.

Your first exercise is *Lunges*. You will be working pretty much every muscle from the waist down, but mostly your butt and thigh muscles. Use a nearby wall to balance with only if you need to. Using a wall instead of a chair or table is important because you won't be tempted to grab onto it to help you with the exercise. You will only be able to use it for balance.

Your front knee should be directly over or behind your front ankle at all times. Never let your front knee go in front of your ankle, as this will unnecessarily load your knee joint and unload your leg muscles. Keeping your front knee back will also work your hamstrings and butt muscles more effectively.

Start with your back knee on the ground and lunge upwards creating 7 complete stops on the way up and 7 stops on the way down. When you reach the bottom of the range, stop just shy of the back knee touching. The only time the back knee should touch should be to start, and when you are finished after reaching full fatigue.

You will begin to lose your balance as you near full fatigue, and when you do reach fatigue, start your holds and work through your pulses. You will find balance increasingly difficult but this is normal and it just proves you are getting to the fatigue necessary. You know you are done with your splinters when you can no longer keep your back knee off the floor.

As muscle fibers fatigue, they stop working. As you push through this fatigue, fewer fibers are available to help with control and balance until finally, you don't even have enough left to keep you off the floor. That is the point where your muscles are shown they have to change because they can't do it!

The picture below shows all seven stops on the way up. Use the same stopping points on the way down. Notice how the top of the range is never achieved and the bottom of the range is cut short an inch so the back knee never touches. This creates the constant tension for faster fatigue mentioned earlier.

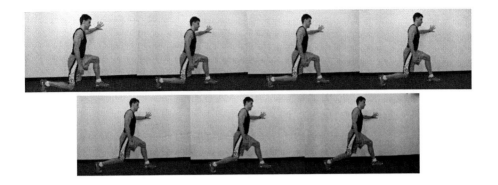

Your second exercise is *Pushups*. You are working chest, triceps, and the front of your shoulders with this exercise. You also are working core muscles, so perfect form is important. Swaybacks and saggy posture take away from the effectiveness and muscle isolation which will cause the set to drag itself out longer than necessary, so stay with the form, especially when you are at full fatigue!

Start with pushups from the hips. This will be less resistance and will allow you to progress up to the knees when strong enough to do 7 perfect reps from the hips. Pushups from the feet are the next step when you can do 7 reps from the knees. If 7 perfect reps are possible from the feet, increase the difficulty by placing your feet up on a chair and keeping your hands on the floor. When doing pushups from the knees or feet, make sure your body is completely straight with absolutely no bending at the hips or swaybacks!

This exercise is a smaller range than lunges, so the 7 stops will feel closer together. On this exercise, lightly touch your chest to the floor at the bottom and stop just shy of locking your elbows at the top. When you touch your chest to the floor, be sure to touch only lightly so the muscles maintain tension and keep working by holding your weight for resistance.

When you hit the wall and can't move any more, hold there until you start to sink to the floor. Then pulse as long as possible until you end up on the floor. Really try to drag this out as long as possible because the longer you spend at fatigue, the faster you will progress. Every second counts exponentially at this point, so pushing yourself that extra few seconds beyond what you think you are capable of will be worth much more than you may realize! The extra effort really will be worth it!

A long touch, bounce, or rest (even ¼ second) will only unload the muscles and prolong the exercise longer than necessary. Locking your elbows at the top will cause the same problem, as the joints take all the pressure and the muscles get to rest. Remember that any rest at all is working against your end goal of failure. A quick rest might feel good at the time and even allow you to keep going with a new sense of energy, but that's not the point. Failure is the point, and the only way your muscles will change, so constant loading and tension are vital to achieving this full fatigue.

Once you reach fatigue, perform your hold and pulse splinters until you can no longer stay off the floor. If you can do 7 perfect reps, go back down to the mid point of the range (halfway between the top and the bottom) and do your holds and pulses there until you end up on the floor.

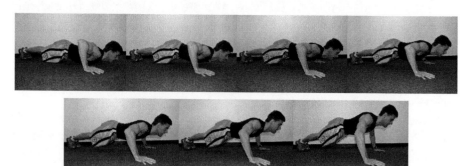

Your third exercise is called *Superhero flyes*. This exercise will work your back, butt, and posture muscles as well as your rear shoulder muscles. Lie on your stomach with your arms in front like superman. Slowly raise your hands straight up and look forward. Your feet will come off the ground as well, but only a few inches. Since this is a very small range, only 4 stops are necessary in both directions. Add an extra pause at the top and stick a quick squeeze in there so you are sure you are at full range.

When you can do 7 reps in good form, try it with some soup cans or books of the same weight in your hands. One to two pounds is all you will need to take yourself to the next level. Remember your holds and pulses at the highest possible point when you get to fatigue or 7 reps. You will know you are at fatigue because you will not be able to get as high as your first rep.

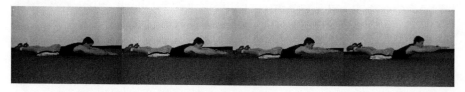

Once you have finished your splinters for superman flyes, move your arms straight out to the side like batman. Now perform the same straight up and down motion with this new posture. Your feet will come off the ground about as high as they did with superman flyes. Follow all the same tips as mentioned above, with special attention to the extra squeeze at the top of the range.

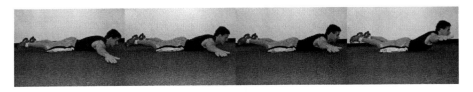

When you have finished your splinters for batman flyes, move your hands and arms down by your sides like aquaman. This will engage your larger and stronger lat muscles in your back, so holding books or soup cans in your hands might be necessary for added resistance.

As you arch up bringing your feet off the floor, raise your hands straight up as far as they will go. If you can reach past your own body, add the extra squeeze at the top by coming together with your hands and trying to touch them behind you. Don't worry if your body is not built this way or you cannot reach your hands together. Try anyway and you will be accomplishing the same peak contraction. After you reach fatigue or 7 perfect reps, finish with your holds and pulses as high as you can keep your hands.

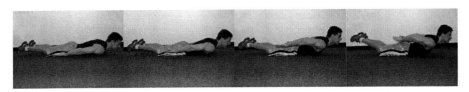

Now roll to your back for *Crunch Twists*. This will train all four layers of your abdominal muscles. Lie flat on your back with your fingers interlaced behind your neck. Your hands are only there to support the weight of your head so keep your elbows wide, and avoid pulling up with your hands. This pulling temptation will increase with your fatigue level, so be constantly mindful of this.

Point your chin to the ceiling and keep it up through the entire range. This will help prevent pulling your head up and forward as well. You can also concentrate on pressing the tip of your tongue to the top of your mouth as an added technique to keep your head in the correct position.

Next, suck your stomach in as far as you can. Visualize pulling your navel to your backbone. Maintain this contraction through the entire range to exercise your deepest stomach muscle called the transverse abdominus. This muscle is responsible for the flat stomach look, so strengthening it is vital to a more toned waist as well as adding strength to your core.

Now crunch up slowly, completing four stops (ratchets) on the way up. Try to get your shoulder blades off the floor, but keep your low back down. When you get to the top of your range, hold it there and twist 4 times back and forth. Each twist should take about 2 seconds each way. Then crunch down slowly, stopping 4 times on the way down as well. You should still be maintaining the "sucking in" you started with. Keep this tension constantly no matter where you are in the range and regardless of the rep you are on.

When you get to the bottom, immediately start back up to your next rep without any pause or rest. The stomach muscles should remain tight the whole time so they fatigue as fast as possible. Taking little breaks or rests will only cause you to have to do more to get to fatigue. It will also rob you of the benefits of the combined strength and endurance this program is designed to deliver.

Go until you reach full fatigue and cannot complete the full range and more. Then hold as high as you can until you start to sink down. At this point, pulse until you can no longer keep your shoulder blades from touching.

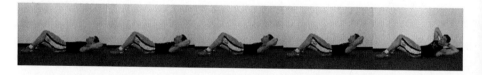

This concludes your starter program! Done correctly, this routine should take you 12-15 minutes to complete. Resting only 1-2 minutes between exercises will increase your cardio as well. Longer rests will still improve your strength but will detract from your cardio improvement.

Performed twice a week, this routine can be done for up to 4 months before your body adapts to it, but research shows that after 6-7 weeks, your brain will need a change. Switching programs every 6-8 weeks also encourages new enervation phases, which continues nerve training, new muscle strengthening, and coordination improvements. Restarting the enervation phase also prevents muscle bulking, so switching every 7 weeks keeps you lean and toned, over big and bulky.

Be sure to stretch when you are done with this or any other strength or cardio routine. Each stretch should take 30-90 seconds, depending on the time you have available. Stretch only to the point of a healthy feeling in the muscles and never past that to where you feel pain. Pushing a stretch too far will cause your muscle to contract in order to protect itself, and will not give any additional flexibility benefits. Research shows that stretching while warm after a strength training workout will add another 10% or more to your strength gains, so this little amount of extra time is worth it!

THE MID STOPS METHOD

Will Rogers once said, "Even if you are on the right track, you'll get run over if you just sit there." This applies to fitness as well as many other things in life! Even though the ratchet protocol is a great method, its problem is that it is just one method. You need to change your method and exercises every seven weeks to keep your nerves changing, your mind learning, and your muscles strengthening.

This method calls for a 4 second pause in the middle of each range. Instead of stopping 7 times on the way up and 7 times on the way down, you are now stopping only in the middle of each rep and for a full 4 seconds.

This routine will require a set of dumbbells and an exercise ball. You can purchase a full set of dumbbells or an interchangeable style if storage space is a consideration. A set that goes from 2 lbs. to 20 lbs. is all you will need unless you are some kind of monster, because all of the protocols in this book necessitate light weights because of the form, exercise style and speed control. An exercise ball can be found at a variety of stores ranging from exercise shops to drug stores. The standard size is fine for most body frames.

Remember to always warm up first so that you are stronger for your workout! According to the research, taking this extra 3-5 minutes gains you an extra 15% or more in overall results. The warm up also adds an important safety factor which makes it harder to "tweak" something or pull a muscle during a workout. Warming up will make you less sore the next day as well, so there are lots of reasons for this short little step!

Your first exercise is hamstring curls. Most people have a natural imbalance between their hamstrings and their quadriceps (thighs), so starting with the hamstrings while your energy is fresh helps to correct this problem. Many knee injuries could be prevented by putting hamstring strength first and emphasizing it properly to match the quadriceps strength.

Your hamstrings should be about 70% as strong as your quadriceps for minimal knee strength and joint stability. An ideal strength ratio would be 1:1, but rarely can you find someone with hamstrings as strong as their quadriceps. Certain competitive skiers and sprinters who train properly have muscle balances approaching 1:1, and also have the fewest knee injuries to match.

Hamstring curls start with your back on the floor and your calves on the ball. Bring your hips up off of the floor to create a straight line from your shoulders to your knees. Maintain this line as you bend your knees and pull your feet in toward your rear. Make a complete 4 second stop on the way up. And then go until you get in as far as you can go.

At this point, your hips will also be at their highest point, because you have been raising them higher through the range to maintain the straight body line from your shoulders to your knees. Keep the hips high at the beginning as well, so you still maintain the straight body posture at all times.

When you reach fatigue, hold and then pulse until your back ends up on the floor. If you reach 7 reps, hold at the apex of the movement where your feet are closest to your butt. Then pulse when you find holding impossible. Continue pulsing until you end up on the floor.

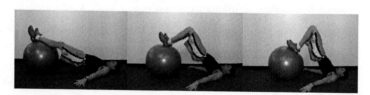

Your second exercise is wall squats. Place your exercise ball between you and the wall, with it placed in the small of your back. As you squat straight down, the ball will roll up your back. You can do this in a corner for added stability if needed. Keep your back straight the whole time and parallel to the wall for the entire range. Make sure you perform a complete 4 second stop at the halfway point on the way up as well as on the way down.

There is no need to stop at the top or the bottom of the range with this protocol. In fact, that will only take away from your results because it can cause opportunity for an offload. Keep constant motion through the top and the bottom of the range, and only stop at the mid points of the range.

Put a box or short stool underneath you to catch you at fatigue, so you don't end up on the floor. Pick something you can sit down on that takes your thighs just below parallel when your butt touches it so it won't interfere with your full range of motion. When you find yourself at fatigue, hold as long as you can, and then pulse until you end up on the box or stool because you are too fatigued to hold yourself off it.

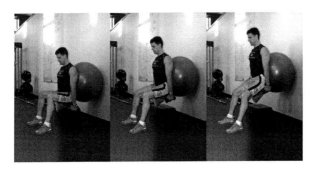

Your third exercise is chest flyes. Lie on top of the ball with wide feet for stability. Your upper back and head should both be on the ball and your low back should be in the air. You might feel unstable, but this is normal and will go away as your nerves get used to the ball.

Start with your arms straight out to the side and pick a dumbbell that is lighter than you think you need (5-12 lbs.) Keep your elbows slightly bent through the whole range. You will be tempted to bend them more as you go down, but make sure they stay only slightly bent.

Stop at the mid point on the way up, and limit your range at the top so you stop before your hands get over your shoulders. This will keep constant tension on your chest and shoulder muscles. Going too far up will cause the muscles to get a rest as the shoulder and elbow joints take the load instead. Going too far down and letting your arms rest on the ball will give another unnecessary rest and cause the exercise to take much longer than necessary to get to fatigue. Remember your hold and pulses when you hit the wall and get stuck on the way up.

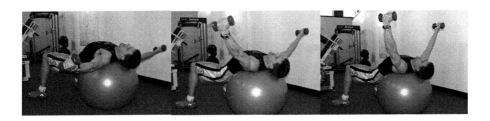

Your fourth exercise is back flyes. This is the same as chest flyes but in reverse with your face down towards the floor. Your arms can stay straight on this one, but make sure you keep them off the ball so you aren't resting at the bottom of each range. The weight you choose should be about half that of your chest flyes weight.

The motion should be straight up and down from the floor, with your arms straight out from your ears at the top. You will have the tendency to come backwards toward your hips as you rise up, but this is only because your body wants your large lat muscles to do the work. Your lats will indeed help with this exercise, but it is meant to target the more important posture muscles that need strengthening in your upper back.

Make complete 4 second stops in the middle of the range up and down, being careful to take your time so you don't end up bouncing on the ball. Remember, it's not the number of reps you complete that matters. It's the fatigue you achieve that makes the muscles change and strengthen as rapidly as possible.

Getting wrapped up in reps or ranges only takes away from your end results as the focus is brought off the fatigue itself. Once you hit the wall and become stuck, hold as long as you can through the burn and then pulse until your arms can no longer stay off the ball.

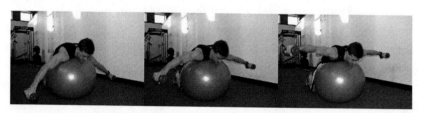

Your fifth exercise is wall curls. Keep your back straight against the wall with your butt and shoulder blades touching at all times. Lock your elbows into your sides and keep them there so your arms don't swing back and forth during the range. Make complete 4 second stops up and down with perfect form, choosing a weight that allows 4-7 reps to complete fatigue.

Be careful to limit your range based on your elbows. If you keep them locked into position at your sides, you won't be able to go high enough to unload your bicep muscles. If you find yourself resting at the top, your elbows have moved forward.

Limit your range of motion at the bottom so your arms are still slightly bent. This will ensure constant tension on your bicep muscles. Your fatigue point and holds will most likely be halfway up or lower, and your pulses should continue until you fail down to the point just above starting with arms slightly bent.

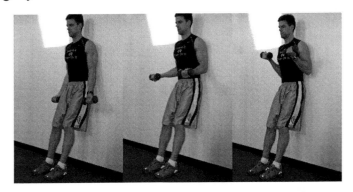

Your sixth exercise is lying triceps extensions. Lying on the floor, grab your dumbbells and start with them just past your head on the floor. Keep your hands apart, but your elbows as close as you can.

Make sure your hands always stay away from the line past your face so that if you were to drop the dumbbells at any point in the range, they would miss your head. This is a great safety factor, but also ensures that constant tension is applied through the entire range.

At the top of the range, your arms should be at a back angle, so when they are straight, tension is still felt on the triceps muscles. At the bottom, stop the range just shy of the dumbbells touching the floor. You will reach fatigue halfway or lower in the range, and your holds and pulses should force your hands back down to the floor.

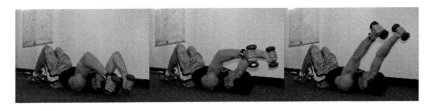

Your seventh exercise is ball crunches. Position yourself as you did with chest flyes, but slightly farther back so that your low back is in contact with the ball. Crunch up with the same form as in the floor crunches of the starter program. This is the same exercise, but will be much more difficult due to the increased range and exaggerated twisting motion made possible by being on the ball.

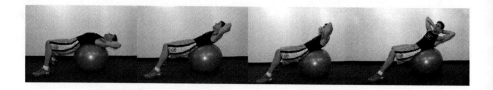

THE TIERED METHOD

This protocol requires you to push up two inches and then down one inch. Every time you go up, stop momentarily as you did with your ratchet method. Then dip down an inch and bounce back up two inches so you get higher with every bounce.

The bouncing activates your stretch reflex which will help you contract more muscle fibers. The controlled stop after the bounce however, keeps it in your nerves as well as your muscles. The small two inch range will prevent high momentum forces from building up, keeping it safe and effective.

When you are ascending, you will push up two inches, stop, then sink down one inch, and bounce up two inches. This "two steps forward and one step back" movement will slowly bring you to the top with 5-7 tiered motions. Be sure to stop before your muscles are relaxed so you are always limiting your range to stay within the constant tension pathway.

The same principle applies on the way back down. Move down two inches and bounce back up one inch, slowly working your way down to the bottom. It sounds more complicated than it really is and may be hard to picture from the photos below, so be sure to go to *www.crackingyourcode. com* to watch the demo video.

Remember to use perfect form. Cheating only cheats you out of isolating the muscles you want to work by involving muscles around them instead. It also prolongs the workout by pushing fatigue further away. You will get done much more quickly and will have more effective results with perfect form.

Failing in perfect form will cause you to hit the wall and get stuck at a certain part of the range. For tiered reps, you may get stuck on the way down as well as the way up, because you may not be able to tier back up the one inch necessary on the return range. That's OK because failure is the whole point, no matter where it happens. Just make sure to include your holds and pulses when you do get to fatigue to round out the process and intensity.

Any of these three methods can be used at home or the gym with any equipment. A bucket of rocks can be just as good for some exercises as a fancy set of machines! Your gym workout routine will vary based on what machines and free weights you have available.

The warm up should be done first with any method or any exercise routine. Stretching afterward is the other activity that adds more benefit than the time it requires. Both the warm up and stretching add a minimum of 10% faster progress EACH, so the time invested is worth the return!

Remember to form a program with the largest muscles first, and move to the smaller muscles second. Your legs, back and chest should always come before your arms so you have maximum energy to use toward the largest muscles. The pictures below demonstrate exercise machines found in most gyms, and beginning range and end range so you can use any method you choose.

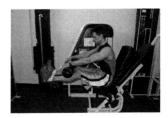
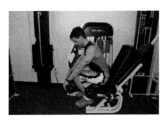

Leg curl start   Leg curl finish

The reason leg curl is listed first (even though it is not the largest muscle), is because most people have an imbalance between their quads and hamstrings. This imbalance can be corrected by putting hamstrings first while energy levels are high. Starting with hamstring exercises also confirms both mentally and physically that this imbalance is a top priority.

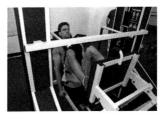
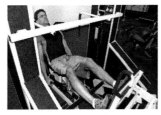

Leg press start   Leg press finish

Notice that the range starts with the weights within an inch of touching and ends with the knees still bent. This prevents unloading the muscle so it never gets a rest. Remember that fatigue is the goal, not completion of a number of reps, so unloading and resting even for a ¼ second will only prolong your set and make your workout take longer to get to fatigue!

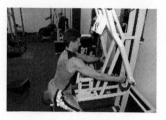
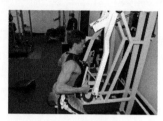

Row start   Row finish

Make sure you keep your chest forward, especially at the end of the range. This will ensure that the angle remains constant and isolation is maximized. If the machine has a chest pad, keep your sternum against it at all times. If it doesn't, do your best to keep the angle constant with your hips so your lower back doesn't do all the work.

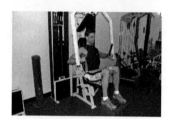
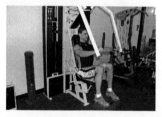

Chest Press start   Chest Press finish

The same rule applies for this pressing motion (and for all pressing motions) as with the leg press. Keep the weights from touching at the bottom and keep your joint from locking at the top for constant tension and maximum fatigue in minimum time!

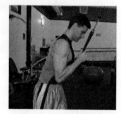
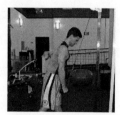

Triceps pushdown start   Triceps pushdown finish

Notice with triceps pushdowns and bicep curls that body position remains constant as well as shoulder angle. This is an isolator exercise with only one joint involved, so any movements of any other joint will only take away from the exercise effectiveness and delay fatigue. Leaning too far forward on triceps pushdowns or too far back on bicep curls also reduces the effectiveness. If you find yourself "cheating" or changing other joint angles for even 1 rep, the weight might be too heavy for you.

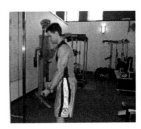
Bicep curl start

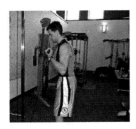
Bicep curl finish

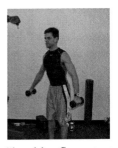
Shoulder flyes start

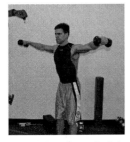
Shoulder flyes finish

The slight forward lean pictured above with both the bicep curl and the shoulder fly, is very important to maintain through full fatigue. This will ensure that you are isolating the proper parts of the muscles. You may have a natural tendency to stand up straight or lean back as you approach fatigue, but succumbing to this temptation completely changes the exercises and will drastically reduce their effectiveness.

Finish with ab crunches as pictured previously on the exercise ball. This will complete your strength routine, but remember to stretch and get your protein when you are done! Your gym will have many different machines, so your health club routine can be quite varied. Just make sure you are changing your exercises and method every 7 weeks for optimal strength gains and minimal plateaus.

CHAPTER SIXTEEN

CRACKING YOUR CORE STRENGTH CODE

Out of every $11 spent on medical care in 2005, according to a new study in the *Journal of the American Medical Association*, $1 of it was for our backs. After adjusting for inflation, *bad backs rang up $86 billion worth of medical expenses* in 2005. That's a 65 percent jump from 1997. On average, expenses for an individual with a back problem added up to $2,580 more in 2005 than for someone without one. Between 1997 and 2005, the cost of pain drugs and other back-related medications almost tripled according to a recent article in *U.S. News & World Report*.

Most adults will have at least one back problem serious enough to see a doctor about. Most back problems can be solved with proper core strength, so the following 5 minute extra credit routine can not only solve your back pain issues, but prevent them from ever coming back!

This routine can be done every day. It is not a muscle failure routine, so sweat and fatigue are not necessary components. I do mine while watching TV or as a quick break from sitting at the computer. You can do just one exercise at a time also. They need not be linked together as a routine to give you the benefit you are after.

Use any one of the three protocols. You can even pick a different one every time. Since you aren't progressing in weight, and just training your core, protocol choice doesn't matter.

The first exercise is called **kneeling crossovers**. Our own X Gym member Krissy, pictured below, is using dumbbells because her core is so strong, but using just using the weight of your hands and feet will most likely be enough. A knee pad is also pictured here, but performing the exercise on a carpet or using a pillow should be sufficient for comfort.

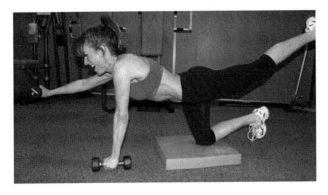

Start with both hands and knees on the ground. Raise your opposite hand and leg (i.e. right hand, left leg) at the same time according to protocol and return to the ground. Then do the same thing with the other arm and leg. Repeat at least 10 times each side, but longer if you have time. This works the deep spinal and posture muscles as well as your nerves and even your brain for improved core strength and coordination.

The next core exercise is called **side planks**. On the floor, prop yourself on your side with your body suspended between your feet and your elbow. Balance there until you are not struggling to hold position. Any protocol can be used, but for ratchets and tiered, it will be only 4 movements instead of 7 because of the small range.

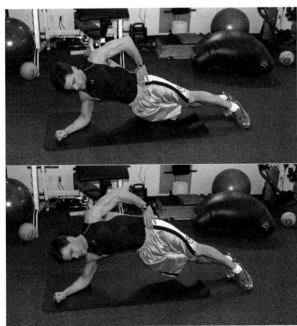

Bottom

Top

You will know you are at fatigue because you can no longer hold a straight posture line from your feet to your head. At this point, hold until you start to sag, and then pulse until you can no longer control the bend and begin to sink to the floor. Repeat on the other side.

Front planks are also a great core exercise, but can easily be done with the wrong form, and hurt your back. For this reason, I recommend just going back to one of the ab exercises previously listed. These will work your deep muscles as well as your surface muscles, so core training will still be maximized.

CHAPTER SEVENTEEN

CRACKING THE AGE AND EXERCISE CODE

The most exciting thing about age and strength training is the research. Until the 70's we thought the older you were, the harder it would be to get strong and build muscle. Thanks to scores of scientific studies since then, we have learned that age has nothing to do with it!

Scientists even compared groups of 20 year olds to groups of 80 year olds and found that with the same intensity level changes, both groups shared the same strength gains and muscle mass increases. Muscles don't know how old they are. Only minds get weaker with age because we let them.

Strength training is one of the only ageless sports. All other sports like football, baseball, basketball, and even running take a toll on the body, and after a while, the "old guys" just can't keep up anymore. 35 years old is retirement age for most professional sports!

The good news is that strength training with weights is very different. Muscles aren't even mature until your 30's, so things are really just getting started then. I've known strongman competitors in their 50's and natural bodybuilders in their 60's who look twice as good as competitors half their age.

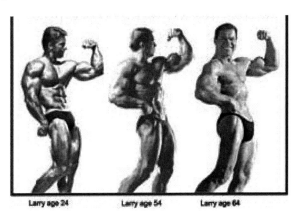

Larry age 24   Larry age 54   Larry age 64

Larry Scott, pictured here, was the first Mr. Olympia bodybuilding champion back in 1965 before steroids hit the scene. As you can see, he looked even better at age 54 than age 24, and at age 64 still had a physique better than 99.9% of the young studs half his age.

Jack LaLanne is another good example of what drug-free strength training and clean living will do for you. At the time of this printing, Jack is still clipping along well into his nineties, doing things most 30 year olds wouldn't even try! At age 70, Jack demonstrated his amazing swimming and cardio endurance by towing 70 boats with 70 people 1.5, miles fighting strong winds and currents the entire way. Oh yeah, and he was handcuffed and shackled to make it more of a "challenge."

As soon as you start saying, "I'm too old for that," or slowing down your pace of life, you will get weaker and turn yourself into an old person. If you refuse to give in and stay active instead, you will maintain your youthful metabolism and vigor just like Jack.

Our cells are replacing themselves constantly. Some cells are even replaced with new ones on a daily basis. Others take months, but within a year, most of your body has been completely regenerated. The main reason people look less healthy year after year and age prematurely is because they are growing new cells based on unhealthy habits. The main reason our metabolisms decrease is because we don't grow new muscle cells to replace the ones we naturally break down!

As humans, we should lose no more than two percent of our metabolism per decade after the age of 40. This means if we don't let ourselves slow down, our metabolism should only have declined 10 percent by the age of 90!

I can even go one better than this. Since my protocols and theories so far have shattered all the scientific evidence, I'm willing to state that I will maintain 95 percent or more of my metabolism when I am 90. I am 41 now, and have the metabolic testing equipment to score mine, so those of you who are still around in 50 years can ask me how I did!

CHAPTER EIGHTEEN

CRACKING YOUR BULKING CODE

Some people come to me asking how to bulk up. While I do know the best ways for this, my emphasis is on strength and tone. You will not bulk up from the methods and protocols in this book, so if you think you are, think again and look at some other factors which I will explain in this section.

There are four levels of fibers that have been identified, but for practical purposes we'll divide them into two: fast twitch fibers and slow twitch fibers. Fast twitch can double in size or even more, if your genetics allow. Slow twitch fibers have a much more limited capacity for size increase and typically top out at about 20% over their original size. Slow twitch fibers are actually better at decreasing their circumference than increasing it, and fast twitch are better at increasing their circumference.

Since slow twitch fibers are the endurance type, they can easily be trained that way. They run on oxygen for fuel, so as they become more efficient aerobically, they get smaller to bring the surface capillaries carrying oxygen closer to the nucleus for processing. This size decrease can be seen among any world class marathon runner.

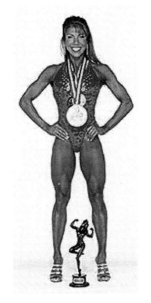

Fast twitch fibers are the power and quick energy fibers so they operate without oxygen (anaerobically). They run on phosphates as fuel and don't need oxygen, so instead of bringing the capillaries closer to the nucleus, they can expand the other way and increase their strain and contractile forces by getting thicker.

Researchers have found that type II muscle fibers have a regulating factor on whole body metabolism through their ability to alter the metabolic properties of other tissues. Since strength training to failure is the best way to build type II

171

muscle fiber, metabolic alterations are most likely through this type of training.

Researchers are currently identifying the novel proteins in muscle that communicate with other tissues. These new proteins, referred to as "myokines" from the Greek words "muscle" and "motion," may represent new targets for therapies that mimic the benefits of weight training for the treatment of obesity and diabetes as well as muscle wasting disorders.

If you are a woman, it simply isn't possible to "bulk up" with two 20 minute sessions per week. It's just not enough time and you don't have the hormones necessary for it anyway. Testosterone is the main hormone responsible for muscle mass and girth increase. Men have this in abundance, so it's easier for them. Some men are bulky and strong without even lifting weights because they have such high levels, but that gift usually comes at the expense of hair loss-another effect of high testosterone.

Women have about the same testosterone levels as a 10 year old boy, so "bulking" is obviously not a possibility. Even women who *want* to bulk cannot do so without the aid of drugs, steroids, excessive supplementation, and hours per day of heavy conventional weight lifting.

Women who *do* spend hours working out and lifting weights *without* the drugs and steroids end up looking like fitness champions like Suzie Curry pictured previously. When Suzie won her second consecutive world championship victory, she reported that her workouts were a "full time job." Exercise *is* her occupation.

Suzie lifts weights *more than 20 hours a week* and trains with cardio another 10-15 hours on top of that! As you can see in her picture, all this exercise has not made her a giant bulky woman. She stands 5 2", weighs 110 lbs. and has a 24 inch waist. Her muscle definition is obvious, but her arms measure only 10.5 inches in circumference. Hopefully you can also understand that if *she* can't bulk up with great genetics and 30+ *hours* of exercise a week, neither will you, on much less workout time, with the anti-bulking methods in this book.

Every woman who has ever come to me feeling as if she were "bulking up" was also dealing with excess weight she needed to lose. She mistakenly assumed that her clothes were getting tighter because of muscle increase instead of fat gain. Women who *gain* weight following an exercise program are doing so because their food intake is increasing (whether it be conscious or not), at a higher rate than they are burning it off.

The protocols in this book are specifically designed to improve strength *without* bulk or weight gain. The constant variation in exercises *and protocols* every seven weeks encourages renewing muscle innervation improvements, but limits the time and repetition necessary for hypertrophy, and effectively skips this phase.

When I was trying to bulk up, my scale weight went up only three pounds in seven months but my *measurements* didn't increase. They all stayed the same or went down because I *traded* fat for muscle. My arms and chest *looked* bigger because of definition improvement, but the girth measurements were the same. My testosterone levels are right in the middle of the normal range for males.

If you are a woman who you feels like you're "bulking up," then your testosterone levels would have to be much higher than an average male's and unless you're growing hair on your palms and could sing bass for the Oakridge boys, that's simply not the issue.

It's easier to blame weight gain on external factors than it is to make the necessary changes to a nutrition program. The question I ask women who are gaining weight at the X Gym is, "do you think exercise is fattening?" They of course answer "no." My next question is, "then what in your life *is* fattening?" If you are gaining weight, or feeling like you are bulking, ask yourself the same question, because it is certainly not due to muscle size increase.

I have also talked with women who feel they have bulked up in the past and are afraid of it happening again. Again, in **every** case, each individual was dealing with a weight issue at the time and misinterpreted their spot-bulking as muscle when it was really fat tissue. Not all women store fat in the same places. Some gain in the arms and shoulders before the hips and thighs and attribute it to muscle bulk. Others gain in the upper back and neck and feel their "traps are bulking up." In all my years as a personal trainer, I have yet to hear a complaint from a lean woman who feels she's bulking up, but have heard the complaint from *dozens* of women who have excess weight they are trying to lose.

The last woman I consulted with was eating a certain food item that was contributing an extra 50 grams of carbs and 30 grams of fat each day without her realizing it, because she had read the label wrong. As soon as she cut it out of her diet, she lost weight at a rate of about two pounds a week! Another woman was doing most of the things right except water consumption. She was chronically dehydrated without knowing it. As soon as she got up to her required intake, she lost the weight and also cured her daily headaches! Take some time and figure out what is fattening in your life. It may even be a habit or practice that you are completely unaware of that is the problem!

If you do want to bulk up, it will take you extra time. You will also have to do more homework than those who are just looking for tone, definition and condition. I won't spend too much time on bulking, because that's not what this book is about, but following the principles and protocols in this book will certainly tone, strengthen and shape your body while drastically reducing the time you have to spend in the gym.

Muscular hyperplasia, or the multiplication of muscle cells, was once thought impossible in humans. This is very interesting to bodybuilders who do want to bulk up because they can increase the size and number of their cells.

New research has found that it is indeed possible, and can even be trained for it. The most recent indications suggest that heavy negative training after eccentric failure is achieved causes some muscle cells to split into two cells.

This was once thought impossible because the new cell has to come up with its own nucleus, mitochondrion, and other cell micro units, but studies have found that the body is actually able to find a way to do this. It was first discovered in bird studies but since then has been proven in humans as well. It is still a mystery how this happens, but is quite exciting none the less!

Fat cells were once thought to multiply only in the womb and during the first year of life, but recent discoveries have found that this is untrue as well. Until recently, we believed that after the first year of life, we had a finite number of fat cells and they just increased in size as we got fatter. Much to our dismay, we found that fat cells can multiply if pushed hard enough, but the good news is they can also die off if unused for long periods of time.

This is bad news for those gaining fat, but good news for those losing fat and more importantly, for those keeping it off. Fat cells will only multiply as a last resort. Only obese people who continue to gain fat rapidly can cause this to happen. This is often referred to as a component in Metabolic Syndrome X and is caused by people who continually hammer away at their set point until it finally gives in and lets them rapidly gain additional fat beyond this set point. At this point, the body has been taught how to essentially ignore the set point, and getting back down is much more difficult.

Metabolic syndrome goes both ways however. Resetting your set point to a lean status will make you more resistant to fat gain and helps you lose it faster when you do gain it. When you get lean and stay lean, fat cells die off, and as you reset your new lean set point, you do so with fewer cells! This metabolic syndrome becomes stronger the longer you stay at your set point, whether it be fat or lean, and the more lean tissue you have, the more likely you will maintain your lean set point. This is why strength training is so important to not only get to your lean set point, but to stay there as well!

Keeping your new set point with fewer fat cells means "cheating" during the holidays has less effect. As long as you stay relatively lean, you won't recreate those cells either. To get them back would take going back to the obese extreme. It's only at the edges of the extremes that we lose or gain the numbers of fat cells we have.

A special note should be made for those who are trying to gain muscle but are vegetarians. Your progress will depend on what type of vegetarian you are. Some people call themselves vegetarians because they eat everything but red meat. This program will work just as well as a "meat eater." Others stay away from all meat but will eat eggs and milk products. This nutrition style will make it a little more challenging to get the proper amounts of protein, but will work just fine with some commitment.

True vegans eat only vegetables and fruits. There is no way to get the proper balance of macronutrients for both gaining muscle and staying lean, so this group must settle for slower results and a very different end goal than their omnivorous friends.

I'm not bashing vegans; I'm just saying we will never see a true vegan on the cover of Men's Fitness or Oxygen magazine. To achieve the muscle needed for obvious definition as well as the low body fat to show it, you must have animal protein.

CHAPTER NINETEEN

CRACKING YOUR CARDIO CODE

Cardio exercise is the icing on the cake. The two 20 minute strength workouts in this book will also provide cardio fitness, so you really are getting both at the same time. Most of the clients at the X Gym don't do any cardio and still enjoy fantastic results from their 2 sessions of strength training per week.

I'm not trying to discourage you from doing cardio, I'm just saying it is extra credit. It will contribute more fat burning and will even help you recover between your strength workouts to augment results there. Cardio exercise will push you further and give you faster results, so it just depends on how much time you have and if that extra effort is worth it to you.

Just like strength training, cardiovascular exercise is all about the intensity. Interval training is your fastest way both to aerobic fitness and fat loss. No longer are you doomed to long duration workouts, because interval training is a huge time saver as well. A 20 minute session can elevate your fat burning rate for 4 hours after you are done with the exercise! Regular cardio typically has only a one-to-one fat burn ratio, which means you will only get an hour's worth of extra fat burning for an hour long session.

Here is how it works. Short maximal bursts activate your fight or flight mechanism because your muscles think you are running for your life. Your body thinks you have moved to a place where there are lots of tigers and bears, so it responds by trying to make you lighter and faster. The fat drops off to make you quicker, and the muscle increases to make you faster. It is a very basic response, but is quite effective and complements your strength training routine as well.

The proper way to do interval training is through maximal effort short burst segments followed by recovery intervals. The most important part of the workout is the short sprint segments, so make sure they really are as fast as you can go.

The recovery intervals in between are just a way to get you ready for the next sprint segment, so make sure you slow down enough to be ready for the sprint. Being recovered will allow you to put 100% into that sprint segment, and that is the most important part.

This recovery time requirement will decrease as your fitness level increases, and your sprints will be easier to accomplish as well. Maximal effort is relative however, so as you become in better shape, your output will increase automatically.

The goal with interval training is to get your heart rate and breathing rate as high as possible during your sprints, and as low as possible during your recovery segments. Graphed on paper, this will show peaks and valleys. The peaks should be as high as possible and the valleys as low as possible. The space between your peaks and valleys will also increase with fitness.

Any change up or down is a good stress on your heart and lungs. Interval training is the fastest way to create this change. The more changes you can fit in, the better your workout will be for fat burning and cardio improvement.

When you first start the program, begin with 10 second sprint intervals and go for a total workout time of 10 minutes. Begin with a two minute warm up at a relatively slow speed that is fairly easy. When your clock hits two minutes, sprint as fast as you can for 10 seconds. Then slow down to recovery speed until the clock hits four minutes. Your 10 minute workout should look like the table below. A graph of your heart rate and breathing rate will look similar to the chart as well:

0:00-2:00 warm up speed
2:00-2:10 sprint
2:10-4:00 recovery speed
4:00-4:10 sprint
4:10-6:00 recovery speed
6:00-6:10 sprint
6:10-8:00 recovery speed
8:00-8:10 sprint
8:10-10:00 recovery speed

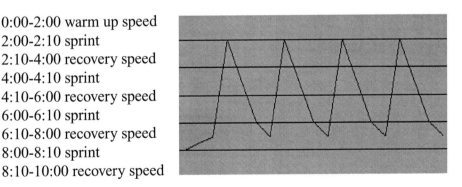

It is very important to make sure you are truly sprinting for the full 10 seconds. That doesn't sound like much time, but if you are doing it right, you won't be able to go more than 10 seconds each sprint and you will be good and ready to be done at the end of the 10 minute workout.

The next time you work out, try 11 second sprint intervals and go for a total time of 11 minutes. Keep increasing each time at this scale until you reach a max of 20 second sprints for 20 minutes. If you get to a certain time frame (i.e. 14 sec. sprints with 14 min. total time) and find it too hard, just stay there until you can do it before you progress to the next level. Pushing yourself to the next level too soon will only make you hate it and form negative nerve pathways in your brain that will turn you away from this type of training.

I must stress again that for this to work; the sprint segments must be truly maximal and exhausting. If you find yourself hitting the wall before your total exercise time is up, just cool down and stop. No big deal. You might be having a bad day or stress might be sapping your energy. Just progress at your own rate until you can do the whole 20 minutes. Even a 10 minute workout can have a metabolic elevation of more than an hour afterward, so do what you can and build from there.

If you are not recovering enough between sprints or aren't pushing yourself fully during sprints, your peaks and valleys will be too shallow and the fat burning effect afterward will be drastically reduced. This is why interval training is best done on a machine that can react fast as your speed changes. Elliptical machines, stationary bikes and running or biking outside are good examples. Treadmills change speed and incline too slowly and stair machines often require the user to adjust the step frequency on the console manually.

It should also be noted that swimming is a crummy way to burn fat. Scientists are still trying to figure out why, but even studies with subjects riding stationary bikes on the pool deck compared to in the pool water had different fat loss results. It is also nearly impossible to do maximal interval training in a pool unless you are a very skilled swimmer with perfect breathing technique.

Now here is the good news. As you become better conditioned, you will actually have to train less! Since you will be able to push yourself harder, you can achieve the same cardio results with progressively less time. I never do more than 8 minutes anymore and am still improving my cardio fitness!

With traditional cardio training, you must exercise longer as your fitness progresses, and continue to push your limits with time instead of intensity. With my present condition, I would have to train at least 2 hours a day with traditional cardio to keep progressing and improving. I sure don't have time for that!

CHAPTER TWENTY

CRACKING YOUR EXCUSES CODE

I have heard the "I'm too busy to exercise" excuse way too often. This book will show you that you only need 20 minutes for a workout, but here are some other tips to save time and squeeze in exercise for busy people on the go.

1.) How much time do you waste at stoplights? Instead of sitting there staring at the light, grab a resistance band and do some inner and outward rotations for your shoulders. I also take advantage of this time by making sure I'm drinking water as I'm waiting for the light to turn green.

2.) Why sit? It is easy to get down on the floor and stretch while you read. You can also reconfigure your computer workstation so you are standing when you are on the computer. Try to avoid sitting whenever possible because it is one of the worst things you can do to your lower back and your metabolism. If you must sit, use an exercise ball instead of a chair so you are at least working your core at the same time. With a ball, you can also take stretch breaks on it and even do abdominal exercises at regular intervals throughout the day.

3.) Have fun in line. Try doing wall sits when you are waiting in line. Put your back against the wall and sink down until your thighs are parallel with the ground or floor. Hold this position as long as you can. If there is no wall nearby, find a partner, touch backs, hook arms and sink down into position.

If others ask you what the heck you are doing, tell them to join in and make a contest out of it. I did this with my kids one day while waiting in line for a movie. When they finally dropped, I had them sit on my lap for added weight until I dropped. We had more fun outside the theater than when we went in, and the people standing in line were certainly entertained as well.

4.) Exercise while you watch TV. My cousin has a rule that he must be doing pushups or sit-ups the entire time during ad breaks. A member at the X Gym lost 5 pounds of pure fat in 2 weeks just by walking on the treadmill the whole time his TV was on.

5.) Roll out of bed and onto your cardio. Not only will you burn more fat at this time of day, but you will also save some time because you won't have to take another shower later to wash the sweat off.

6.) Suck it in. The transverse abdominus is the deepest stomach muscle and is the one most responsible for the "flat" stomach look. When this muscle is toned, your stomach will look and feel much flatter because it is more able to hold in your internal organs and the fat around them (visceral fat).

Most people don't exercise this muscle because they don't know how. Crunches have nothing to do with toning it, and while most people think ab exercises will help bring their stomach in, they are doing them all wrong.

I have seen many people with "washboard abs" while they are flexing them, but when relaxed, their stomach distends. This distention is due to a weak transverse muscle. In the case of professional bodybuilders however, it has more to do with steroids and growth hormone than weak muscles. Anabolic drugs always cause a drastic increase in visceral fat, so the big gut you see on them is from this excess fat pushing out from the inside.

The fibers of the transverse abdominus run sideways across your body so the only way to train them is to suck your stomach in as far as you can. This is most effective to do while doing other ab exercises because the other stomach muscle layers will try to pull it back out.

You can also work the transverse muscles any time and anywhere by simply sucking in. The best way to contract this muscle is to totally relax and let your gut "hag out." Then slowly pull it in until you can't pull any farther. At that point, hold it for 5 seconds while trying to pull even further the whole time. Then slowly let it back out to the start position and begin over. Do this as many times as you like. The more the better, and every day is OK, but if you are sore from a previous session, wait until that goes away so you can fully recover.

I exercise mine while driving in the car. I also work them while standing in line somewhere or any time I feel like I am doing nothing and wasting time. I am usually in loose clothing, but if I am in tighter clothes I do occasionally get strange looks. I just tell them it's the alien moving inside me and they pretty much leave me alone.

7.) Do isometrics anywhere and anytime. Grabbing any immovable object and pulling, pushing, or lifting until fatigue will help strengthen your muscles and build metabolism stoking tissue. Be careful though, because as you get stronger through the methods in this book, you will find previously immovable objects become moveable (or breakable)!

CHAPTER TWENTY ONE

CRACKING THE FITNESS
PLATEAU CODE

Fitness plateaus are why most people give up on fat loss. These plateaus happen with fitness progress as well as weight loss and fat loss. People think progress should always be constant, and when it slows or stops, they just figure it isn't working anymore and give up.

The good news is you don't have to put up with them! If you understand the reason they happen and can recognize the symptoms, this book has a plan to solve this problem and break the perpetual plateaus so that many are frustrated with.

At the beginning of the weight loss process most people lose visceral (internal) fat first, so you might not see much in the mirror right away. You are also gaining muscle because you are eating better and finally absorbing nutrients. Fat is being traded for muscle, which will slow or stop scale changes, so ignore the scale and just go with the way your clothes are fitting to mark your progress.

Weight gain sometimes happens in the beginning of a new diet and exercise program if you are gaining muscle faster than you are losing fat. This is especially true for overweight individuals who are sedentary, but don't let this throw you off because it just means your metabolism is increasing as well.

I have seen many people gain weight while they are losing inches at the same time. This, of course, is puzzling to them, but as soon as they understand the phenomenon and take their focus off of the scale, their stress goes away. A pound of muscle takes up about half the space a pound of fat does, so you can see how trading tissues helps you lose inches even though the scale might not parallel those results.

Fat loss never happens in a straight line because the body wants to make sure you don't starve to death. It will slow fat loss with occasional periods of reduced progress so it has some time to make sure everything is still OK. When it has finished its "system check", it will let you resume your previous fast fat loss.

The people who stick it out during the slow spots end up winning in the end, but understanding them, and not being surprised by them is vital. Once a slow spot hits, that sometimes means a program change is in order. This change could mean a different nutrition approach, tweaking your exercise method, or both.

Some slow spots can be overcome with no changes, so it is important to wait it out for a few weeks to make sure. If a month or more goes by with reduced progress, you can change your plan to fire things up again. Variety is key here because your body will try to adapt in every situation. Even the best diet in the world is only as good as the time it takes for you to adapt to it. The same goes for exercise. The best machine, method or protocol is only effective until you adapt. Then a different approach needs to happen for continued progress.

Some plateaus are created by overtraining. This occurs when nutrition and recovery are insufficient. Following the exercise principles in this book will help ensure you will not be exercising too much, but you still need proper nutrition and rest to be ready for your next workout. If your body is still recovering, and you start another workout, you can have a cumulative effect that can build up over time and just break you down.

Career athletes who work out for a living, can actually give themselves cancer and other diseases from overtraining. Free radical buildup is a normal reaction to intense exercise and should not be a concern, but if intense exercise is too long, too frequent, and with inadequate recovery between sessions, free radicals keep building up without adequate time to break them down, and overtraining or even disease can result.

Severe overtraining will always cause a plateau or decreased progress. People who are overtraining and showing diminished progress often go the other way and just train harder, thinking this will solve the problem, but it just makes things worse. The methods in this book are designed for enough time between sessions and are short enough in duration that free radicals will not accumulate faster than they can be broken down.

Overtraining symptoms are varied, but can include chronic fatigue, lethargy, joint soreness, tendon soreness, chronic muscle soreness, and frequent illness. If you are feeling sick, you probably should not be working out. If you feel achy, have a fever, or have symptoms below your neck, that is probably your body saying it needs all your energy for the immune functions and using that energy for a workout will make things worse. If you are in doubt, leave it out or ask your doctor.

If your muscles are still sore, give them another day of rest. Cardio might be OK, unless the soreness was caused by a cardio workout. Sore muscles are typically telling you they are still in the recovery process and need more time to complete it properly. Use this time to feed them what they need with plenty of water, protein and dark greens.

CHAPTER TWENTY TWO

CRACKING THE REST AND RECOVERY CODE

Proper recovery can be what makes or breaks your program. Proper rest and recovery are vital to getting the most out of your workouts. Exercise breaks the muscle down, and rest and recovery builds it back up. You actually make yourself weaker during your exercise session, but during the time between workouts, your body is building back to where it was and then some to get stronger for the next session.

Proper nutrition and hydration are two vital components to becoming stronger and fitter. Your muscles need adequate building blocks to rebuild stronger than before. This means eating the right foods and in the right amount. Since muscles are 70% water (or more), it is obvious how replenishing their main ingredient will help and how dehydration can stop progress completely.

Protein is the next most important component. When muscles are broken down through high intensity training, little "pockets" are created in the cell that can be filled with new protein. Research shows that ingesting 20-40 grams of protein within 5 minutes of a workout, and then another 20 grams every hour for the next 4-5 hours will maximize filling these "pockets" created from the workout.

For some people, this protocol might be too rigid or hard to implement so I usually recommend 40 grams right before, during or right after the workout, and then more as soon and as frequently as possible. I can't always get 20 grams every hour myself with the busy schedule I hold, so doing the best I can works well enough.

My post-workout source usually comes from a protein shake because I typically am not hungry right after training because high intensity exercise is a strong appetite suppressant. I can drink a shake however. My next sources after that usually come from meat. Sometimes I will fall back on a whole food organic protein bar as a last resort.

Protein is best absorbed by eating dark green vegetables. Dark greens have the vitamins and minerals you need, but also in the right ratios. This balance promotes optimal absorption, whereas junk food blocks it. I have known plenty of people who can't seem to absorb protein because of all the junk foods that get in their way.

Always ask yourself the question, "Is this food going to help me recover?" to help you decide if it should go in your mouth or not. Tell yourself in the morning that you will have a good recovery eating day. Focusing on recovery eating will help you make conscious and unconscious decisions each day to not only make that happen, but also to help you lose fat.

The top recovery foods also happen to be the 7 foods listed earlier that you can eat any time and in any amount. Some of the foods that will break you down and cause over training or slow results are also listed earlier as the foods that will lower your metabolism.

A short warm up before the workout and stretching afterwards will also speed your recovery. The warm up will lubricate your muscles so soreness and inflammation due to internal muscle friction is reduced. Stretching afterward helps flush inflammatory chemicals out of the cell as well (see the flexibility section for specifics on stretching).

It only takes 3-5 minutes for a proper warm up and another 3-5 minutes for a complete stretching routine after to do the job. These 6-10 minutes will augment your strength gains another 20% or more, so it really is worth the time!

Sleep is another necessary component to your recovery program. Your body does most of its rebuilding while you are asleep. During this time, you are repairing problems, growing new muscle, and releasing hormones that create optimal progress in your fitness and fat loss goals. If you are eating good whole foods and staying hydrated, sleeping is the best time to reduce inflammation as well.

Certain phases of sleep cause release of specific hormones necessary for proper balance and health. The two main hormones are cortisol and testosterone. Cortisol breaks down tissue, but is necessary for maintaining balance in the body because cells need to be turned over often for optimal health.

Testosterone on the other hand, builds tissue. Both men and women have these hormones for these important functions. Growth hormone is another major hitter that is released at its peak during the sleep hours. This hormone also rebuilds your tissues and helps combat the effects of aging, so the more the better!

Most people need 7-8 hours of quality sleep per night. Less than 6 hours usually results in too much cortisol and not enough testosterone or growth hormone release. Uninterrupted sleep is very helpful because waking during the night will cut certain sleep cycles short and rob you of those hormone release segments.

Certain occupations and lifestyles aren't suited for more than 6 hours of sleep at a time, so in that case a nap during the day can help you catch up and get to your important sleep phases faster that night. Research shows that naps should last 30-45 minutes only. More than 45 minutes can make it hard to get to sleep at night, and shorter than 30 minutes may give you little to no additional help.

Nutrition is just as important as sleep, if not more. I tell my clients to "eat for recovery" and that often takes care of other nutrition problems at the same time. Sugar, HFCS, preservatives, dehydration, and "junk foods" will all hurt your recovery. Providing cells with clean food that is full of nutrients will make your cells repair themselves and build as fast as possible.

CHAPTER TWENTY THREE

CRACKING THE HOME GYM EQUIPMENT CODE

We certainly aren't hurting for exercise infomercials and marketing companies pushing the latest and greatest workout products. According to them, the only true way to finally achieve your goals is with their product. Those who do get sucked in and make the purchase end up disappointed to say the least and become even more discouraged than before.

Then come the New Year's resolutions. Spouses hoping their partner will make the weight loss promise on January 1st often gift exercise equipment for Christmas. Others buy it themselves making December and January the biggest sale months for all the home gym stores as well as the infomercial vultures.

Most of these machines end up becoming towel drying racks by February and by April, the dust layer on the frame of the machine is irritating your allergies. Even though your use of the machine has stopped, your intentions are still to start up again once you get "more time" because you just became "so busy." There it sits for another few months as a reminder of another failed stab at getting in shape. Spring cleaning time rolls around and it ends up being posted on eBay or set out in your front yard with a "Free-take it" sign taped to the front.

All you really need for strength training is a set of dumbbells and an exercise ball. Your minimal requirement for cardio is even less. Just go outdoors! Interval training on a nearby track or even your street is pretty easy to do, and certainly the cheapest way to go. If you live in a cold or wet climate or must purchase a machine, make sure you are mentally ready to commit, and buy something that will last. This will cost more money, but will be worth it later on.

The best place to go for cardio equipment is a specialty exercise store that only sells workout equipment. A good elliptical machine or treadmill will usually cost $1700-3000 and a spinning bike will be $800 or more. Try it out at the store before you buy to make sure it has a good movement pattern for your body frame.

I prefer whole body exercise equipment like an elliptical trainer with moving handles, or a rowing machine. Simultaneous upper and lower body muscle involvement will help you get more done in a shorter amount of time. It will also help you get to your target fatigue with interval training faster than with upper or lower body only machines.

The general sports equipment stores sell the cheapest equipment with the shortest warranties. Even though their typical product guarantee lasts 90 days, it will probably wear out sooner than that if you really use it. They are gambling on the fact that you will use it like the average consumer does, which is for 2-4 weeks, and then stop. They purposely build the product to last about 6-8 weeks so it merely outlasts your weak commitment.

For weight training, a set of dumbbells and an exercise ball is really all you need. There are some selectorized dumbbell options that take up less space, and the ball can easily be stored in a closet, so dedicating a whole room for a home gym is not necessary. The best abdominal machine I have found is also the exercise ball, so this can be your most valuable piece of equipment because it will double as a workout bench as well.

CHAPTER TWENTY FOUR

CRACKING YOUR FLEXIBILITY CODE

Why do we get tighter with age? The answer is simple. It is only because we move less and decrease our own active range of motion each day. After we graduate high school, we slow down for college so we can study more. The time spent each day sitting in a chair doubles. After we graduate from college, our time spent being sedentary usually doubles again.

This fourfold decrease in activity saps our energy so we sit more at home too. All this sitting and slowing creates a lifestyle that causes our muscles to tighten up even more. Our joints aren't using the range of motion they used to, and the muscles tighten up accordingly.

Our muscles continue to atrophy from disuse and pretty soon we find ourselves becoming injured from previously harmless movements like reaching for the milk across the table or even throwing our neck out in our sleep! We just chalk it all up to the effects of aging and convince ourselves that's the way it has to be as we get older.

You can reverse a large part of this process by stretching regularly. The best time to stretch is while you are warm because your muscles will be more supple and responsive to flexibility movements. Science has shown that if you stretch while warm and hold stretches while cooling back down, your flexibility will increase even faster.

Stretching after a workout is the absolute best time for flexibility improvement. Stretching before a workout does little to nothing for flexibility and injury prevention like most people believe. Scientific studies have also shown that stretching after your strength training workout will even increase your strength gains by 10% or more over not stretching at all!

If you really want rapid flexibility increases, stretch while you are cooling down after exercise. When you finish your cardio or strength workout, start your stretch while you are still warm. Continuing to stretch as you cool down will increase flexibility permanently instead of just temporarily, like cold stretching or hot stretching.

One of my university professors (Bill) had a shoulder injury that began to show symptoms of "frozen shoulder." This condition happens when range of motion is reduced over time due to pain. This decreased range of motion progresses to the point where the shoulder has such a diminished range, it is classified as frozen shoulder. Frozen shoulder usually only gets worse as adhesions form inside the joint, and painful physical therapy is typically the only solution.

Bill saw this happening and wanted to put a stop to it fast. He went down to the athletic training room and put some moist heat on his shoulder for about ½ hour to thoroughly and deeply heat his shoulder. He took the heat off and put his shoulder into a stretch. Because he was heated, he was able to comfortably stretch his shoulder beyond its normal limits.

He then held this stretch and wrapped his shoulder in an ice pack to cool it quickly. About 10 minutes later, he removed the ice and slowly came out of the stretch. This process gave him an immediate flexibility increase of about 2 months' worth of regular stretching and rehab work.

Regular heat and ice pack treatments are pretty difficult to orchestrate, but regular stretching after a workout as you are cooling down is easy to do. Each stretch should be held for 30 seconds and the total number of stretches should be seven or so for a whole body routine. This takes less than 5 minutes, so adding this to a routine is pretty easy to do for such a huge payback in flexibility improvement and additional strength gains!

There are plenty of trends out there and stretching gizmos that promise superior flexibility results, but good old fashioned static stretching when warm and holding positions while cooling down is the best way to increase flexibility, and the cheapest as well! The only expense is time, and if you do it while watching TV or reading a book, you aren't even wasting that!

A current trend called "hot yoga" is making quite a splash. People think it is effective because while they are in the hot studio atmosphere, they are much more flexible than at home or regular yoga studios. This increase in flexibility however, is only temporary. Since you are hot during class, of course you will be more flexible. The overall flexibility increase however, will be no better than stretching elsewhere.

Hot yoga has some drawbacks as well. You will sweat quite a bit during hot yoga and this loss of fluid can cause serious dehydration or electrolyte imbalances. People sometimes get cramps later on, or headaches from the effects of fluid and electrolyte loss. Dehydration will also make it harder to lose fat for the reasons discussed previously, and will actually reverse most of the flexibility gains you may have received from the class. Dehydrated muscles are tight muscles, and get sore much more easily as well.

Hot yoga classes do have a lower incidence of stretching related injuries because of the increased muscle temperature, but since regular yoga or other stretching has such a low injury rate anyway, the difference is negligible.

Remember that stretching while warm is more effective because you are more flexible, but it's the *stretching while cooling* that is the most effective way to increase flexibility permanently. Hot yoga is only stretching while hot. There is no stretching while cooling component, so save your time and money and stick with your own stretching time after your own workouts for optimal flexibility improvement.

Below are pictures of 7 basic stretches that you can do after your workouts. Be sure to hold each stretch 30 seconds or longer, and stretch both sides for arms and legs (only one side is pictured). It should not feel like work. Just ease into each position and hold in a good stretch, but not to the point of pain.

Stay still and avoid fast movements into or out of position or bounces while you are in position. Your muscles should be relaxed when stretching. If you stretch too far, your muscles will tighten up and you could be making yourself tighter instead of looser! Visualize your muscles relaxing and elongating. You will find that you are able to ease further into a stretch the longer you hold it, as the muscle releases and allows you to go there.

Come out of the stretch as slowly as you go into it. You are trying to help your muscles relax and recover as well as elongate, so treat them gently. If you feel any pain in the muscle, back off to the pain-free point. The same goes for a joint, ligament or tendon. Stretching should always be pain free.

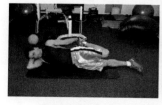 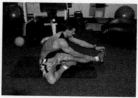 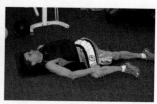

Quad stretch   **Hamstring stretch**   **Hip and low back stretch**

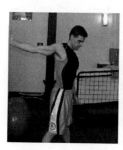 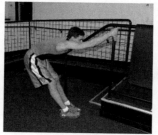 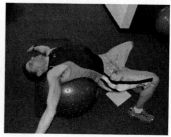

Pec stretch   **Lat stretch**   **Posture stretch** (my favorite)

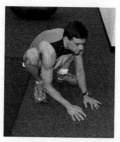

Low back stretch

CHAPTER TWENTY FIVE

CRACKING THE RECIPE CODE

Food preparation, cooking and baking don't have to take lots of time and effort. I hate to cook, and find it a bore, so I have developed the following recipes to be quick and easy. They are also high in the fat burning and protein zones so they should help you lose the fat you want and help you gain muscle at the same time.

Fat Zapping Turkey Meatloaf

Ingredients:

- 1 teaspoon chicken instant bouillon
- 1/2 cup salsa (max 2 net carbs per spoonful)
- 1.5 lbs. lean ground turkey breast
- 1/2 cup oats or Quinoa flakes
- 1/2 cup onion, chopped
- 2 teaspoons basil
- 1/2 teaspoon garlic powder
- 1/4 teaspoon pepper (or lemon pepper for an extra zing)
- 2 egg whites

Cooking Instructions:

- Preheat oven to 350 degrees
- Mix ingredients together and pack into non stick cupcake pan
- Cook for one hour
- Let stand for 10 minutes
- Serve with salsa (3 tablespoons per slice) for an extra kick.
- Each serving is 2 cup cakes
- Makes 6 servings

Nutrient Breakdown:

- One serving has 128 calories
- Fat: 1.5 grams or 11% by calories
- Carbs: 6.75 grams or 21% by calories
- Protein: 21.75 grams or 68% by calories

Fiberilla Burritos

Ingredients:

- 4 oz. ground turkey breast
- 1 Don Pancho low fat/low carb wrap (Safeway)
- Chili seasoning
- 2 tablespoons fat free sour cream
- 1/4 cup shredded fat free cheddar
- 2 tablespoons unsweetened ketchup or salsa
- 2 tablespoons green taco sauce

Note: Ingredients listed are per serving but you will need at least 1 pound of turkey breast to make it worth your while.

Preparation Instructions:

- Cook ground turkey in non-stick pan with 1/4 packet of chili seasoning per pound of meat. Stir and chop constantly, as cooking dry meat with no oil will burn if not attended continuously.
- Spread sour cream in a swath down the middle of the tortilla wrap.
- Put 4 oz. cooked turkey along the same swath.
- Combine the rest of the ingredients, close wrap and chow!

Nutrient Breakdown:

- Each wrap has 298 calories
- Fat: 6 grams or 18% by calories
- Carbs: 24 grams or 17% by calories after net is calculated with a whopping 11 grams fiber factored in!
- Protein: 48 grams or 64% by calories

PJoe's Special

Ingredients:

- 1 pint of Egg Beaters (or other brand egg product in the carton)
- 1/2 cup shredded low fat parmesan
- 3 Morningstar breakfast patties or cooked ground turkey breast
- 4 cups chopped spinach
- 1 tablespoon lemon pepper

Cooking Instructions:

- Spray wok with cooking spray
- Pour egg product into wok and set burner to medium
- Add spinach
- Microwave Morningstar patties for 1 minute on high or use cooked ground turkey breast instead.
- Chop patties and mix in wok (or add cooked ground turkey breast).
- Mix in lemon pepper
- Add parmesan, wait until it starts to melt and serve
- Makes 3 servings

Nutrient Breakdown:

- One serving has 295 calories
- Fat: 14 grams or 42% by calories (or use less parmesan for low fat version)
- Carbs: 8 grams or 11% by calories
- Protein: 35 grams or 47% by calories

Blackjack's Chicken Fajitas

Ingredients:

- 1 lb. organic chicken strips
- 1 red and 1 green bell pepper
- 1/2 cup sliced red onion

- 1 packet of fajita seasoning mix
- 1/4 cup Kraft Fat Free Italian dressing

Preparation Instructions:

- Slice the bell peppers and sauté them with the chopped onion in the Italian dressing until cooked (onion will start to turn translucent.).
- Set veggies aside and cook meat thoroughly with the fajita seasoning mix (following instructions on the mix packet).
- Add the veggies back in and cook together for 3 minutes.
- Serves 4

Nutrient Breakdown:

- Each serving has 168 calories
- Fat: 3 grams or 16% by calories
- Carbs: 9.5 grams or 23% by calories
- Protein: 26 grams or 61% by calories

Harley's Shredded Veggie Bonanza

Ingredients:

- 5 celery stalks (about one bunch)
- 3 handfuls of baby carrots or 2 large carrots
- 1 cucumber
- 1 head of broccoli
- 10 oz. spinach
- 12 oz. cooked turkey or chicken
- 1/2 bottle of *Follow Your Heart* brand low fat dressing (found at PCC or Whole Foods)

Preparation Instructions:

- Slice everything up in your food processor in the order listed above, so when you dump it in the bowl it comes out layered properly.

- Use any other veggies you can think of in place of or in addition to those listed!
- Dump it all in a big ol' Tupperware bowl with the meat on top and pour dressing.
- Serves 4 or just you for a whole day!

Nutrient Breakdown:

- Each serving has 227 calories
- Fat: 4 grams or 18% by calories
- Carbs: 21 grams or 24% (net) by calories
- Protein: 28 grams or 57% by calories

Note: Fiber is **10 grams per serving** with this simple meal and the **vitamin level** can't be beat! If you can make this option a habit the fat will literally **FLY** off of you!

Wilster's Mock Smashed Potatoes

Ingredients:

- 2 tablespoons fat free cream cheese
- 1 medium head of cauliflower
- 1/2 tablespoon minced Garlic
- 1/8 tablespoon salt
- 1/8 tablespoon pepper

Preparation Instructions:

- Cut the cauliflower into small pieces and boil it for 7 minutes. Drain well and dump (while still warm) into food processor or blender.
- Add other ingredients and puree until almost smooth.
- 2 big servings!

Nutrient Breakdown:

- Each serving has 44 calories

- Fat: 0 grams
- Carbs: 4.5 grams or 24% (net due to fiber) by calories
- Protein: 4 grams or 57% by calories

Sony Mac's Turkey Stew

Ingredients:

- 2 lbs. ground turkey breast
- 1/2 red onion
- 3 handfuls baby carrots (or 4 large carrots)
- 1 bunch of celery
- Shelled soybeans
- 1 tablespoon garlic powder
- 1 tablespoon spice of choice
- 1 tablespoon basil
- 1 tablespoon lemon pepper
- 1 cube chicken bouillon dissolved in 4 cups of water (or 8 cups if prepared on stovetop).
- 6 oz. can of tomato paste

Preparation Instructions:

- Chop the carrots and celery (a food processor is fastest).
- Dump everything in a crock pot or stove top pot.
- Cook for 2 hours on high if using a crock pot or 1 hour on medium if stove top. Be sure to check that meat is cooked thoroughly.
- Makes 10 big servings!

Nutrient Breakdown:

- Each serving has 173 calories
- Fat: 3 grams or 15% by calories
- Carbs: 9 grams or 21% by calories
- Protein: 28 grams or 64% by calories

Julio's Taco Salad

Ingredients:

- 1 lb. ground turkey breast
- 3 oz. Kraft fat free shredded cheddar
- 1/4 packet taco seasoning
- 4 tablespoons fat free sour cream
- 7 tablespoons unsweetened ketchup
- 4 cups shredded lettuce
- 1/4 cup chicken broth

Preparation Instructions:

- Cook the ground turkey breast in a pan with the chicken broth (instead of oil)
- Mix in the taco seasoning
- Dump it out of the pan onto the shredded lettuce
- Put sour cream and cheese on top
- Makes 4 servings

Nutrient Breakdown:

- Each serving has 183 calories
- Fat: 1 gram or 4% by calories
- Carbs: 7 grams or 15% by calories
- Protein: 37 grams or 82% by calories

The Captain's Fish Soup

Ingredients:

- 7 tilapia fish fillets
- 2 cups shredded carrots
- 3 cups shredded celery
- 4 cups chicken broth

- 2 tablespoons basil
- 2 tablespoons curry
- 4 cups water
- 1 packet McCormick low sodium taco seasoning
- 1 cup shredded broccoli

Preparation Instructions:

- Put everything in a crock pot or big ol' stovetop pot. cook 3 hours on high for crock pot or 4 hours on medium for stove top pot.
- Makes 10 servings

Nutrient Breakdown:

- Each serving has 120 calories
- Fat: 2 grams or 15% by calories
- Carbs: 8 grams or 16% by calories
- Protein: 20 grams or 69% by calories

Spicy Peanut Bake

Ingredients:

- 5 white fish fillets or 5 chicken breasts (or any other moist white meat)
- "A Taste of Thai" brand *Spicy Peanut Bake* packet.
- Cooking spray
- Baby spinach leaves
- "The Silver Palate" brand *Raspberry Vinegar*

Preparation Instructions:

- Put meat in a non-stick baking tray.
- Spray meat lightly with cooking spray and sprinkle 1 packet Spicy Peanut Bake over meat.
- Bake at 350 for 20-25 minutes (30-40 for frozen meat).
- Spread out baby spinach leaves 2-3 deep on plate and pour 2 oz. raspberry vinegar over them.

- Place baked meat on top of spinach leaves and chow down!
- Makes 2 servings

Nutrient Breakdown:

- Each serving has 406 calories
- Fat: 7 grams or 16% by calories
- Carbs: 17 grams or 17% by calories
- Protein: 68 grams or 67% by calories

Chuck's Texas Meat Balls

Preparation Instructions:

- 1.5 lbs. ground *GRASS-FED* beef
- 1 egg white
- 1/2 cup salsa
- 1 tablespoons garlic powder
- 1 tablespoons "Spike" meat seasoning mix

Preparation Instructions:

- Put all the ingredients in a bowl and mash by hand until thoroughly mixed.
- Roll into balls and put on cookie sheet.
- Bake at 350 for 1 hour.
- Pat meat balls on paper towel to clean and enjoy!
- May also be eaten with salsa or unsweetened ketchup.
- Makes 5 servings

Nutrient Breakdown:

- Each serving has 348 calories
- Fat: 17 grams or 43% by calories
- Carbs: 11 grams or 13% by calories
- Protein: 38 grams or 44% by calories

PJ's Easy Protein Shake

Ingredients:

- 2 scoops MRM brand whey powder (make sure it is the 100% natural variety that is sweetened with Stevia!)
- 1 Quart Organic vanilla soymilk

Preparation Instructions:

- Put all the ingredients in a cup and blend thoroughly with an electric blender
- Chug it down and it revisit your chocolate milk days as a kid!

Nutrient Breakdown:

- Each serving has 556 calories
- Fat: 16 grams or 26% by calories
- Carbs: 39 grams or 28% by calories
- Protein: 64 grams or 46% by calories

Remember that this is a whole quart, so spread it out over a few hours and drink it slowly for best absorption.

Trilster's Blender Bisque

Ingredients:

- 2 fillets cooked Tilapia fish
- 1 cup Chicken broth
- 1 cup nonfat milk
- 1/4 purple onion
- 4 tablespoons shredded parmesan
- 1 teaspoon garlic powder
- 1 teaspoon lemon pepper

Preparation Instructions:

- Blend all the ingredients thoroughly with an electric blender.
- Add a dash of Tabasco for an extra zing.
- Heat in microwave or stove top
- Makes 4 servings

Nutrient Breakdown:

- Each serving has 100 calories
- Fat: 1.75 grams or 16% by calories
- Carbs: 4.25 grams or 17% by calories
- Protein: 17 grams or 67% by calories

Crock Pot Delight

Ingredients:

- 1 GRASS-FED sirloin roast (2 lbs.)
- 1 quart organic chicken broth
- 1 tablespoon garlic powder
- 1 tablespoon Italian spices
- 10 oz. broccoli florets
- 8 oz. baby carrots
- 1 chopped purple onion

Preparation Instructions:

- Pour in broth and add garlic and Italian seasonings
- Add roast
- Place carrots, broccoli and onion around the roast
- Slow cook for 8-10 hours. The longer it cooks, the more tender the meat gets!
- Makes 4 servings
- Great to drink as a nutritious soup as well!

Nutrient Breakdown:

- Each serving has 374 calories
- Fat: 10 grams or 30% by calories
- Carbs: 16 grams or 21% by calories
- Protein: 37 grams or 49% by calories

"Norman on the Foreman" Wrap

Ingredients:

- 1 Don Pancho 36 g wrap (Safeway)
- 2 tbsp. Arriba Salsa (Fred Meyer)
- 2 tbsp. Desert Pepper Black Bean Dip (Safeway)
- 1 Rice Slice tofu "cheese"
- 2 tbsp. fat free Quark
- 3 oz. organic free range, *grass-fed* ground beef

Preparation Instructions:

- Cook ground beef on a Foreman grill
- Spread bean dip on inside of wrap
- Place ground beef, salsa, and Rice Slice on wrap
- Microwave for 14 seconds
- Add Quark, roll shut and enjoy!
- Makes 1 serving

Nutrient Breakdown:

- Each serving has 277 (net) calories
- Fat: 9 grams or 29% by calories
- Carbs: 8 (net) grams or 12% by calories
- Protein: 41 grams or 59% by calories

Fat Furnace Frittata

Ingredients:

- 2 lbs. lean ground beef *ORGANIC GRASS-FED ONLY!*
- 1 package frozen organic broccoli
- 1 package frozen organic chopped spinach
- 1 pint organic egg whites
- 2 tbsp. Spicy (or regular) Mrs. Dash
- 1 tbsp. cinnamon

Preparation Instructions:

- In a HUGE frying pan or 2 regular pans, spray cooking spray and preheat until hot.
- Dump in beef and stir until pink
- Dump in broccoli and spinach and stir with beef until thawed.
- Add spices and egg whites
- Stir until beef and egg whites are fully cooked
- Makes 5 servings.

Nutrient Breakdown:

- Each serving has 637 calories
- Fat: 30 grams or 51% by calories
- Carbs: 30 grams or 3% (net) by calories
- Protein: 62 grams or 46% by calories

Yes, this seems high fat, but the high CLA fat content in the *grass-fed* beef will melt the fat off your body!

Broiled Broccoli

Ingredients:

- 10 oz. frozen organic broccoli
- Salt
- Cooking spray

Preparation Instructions:

- Pour frozen broccoli out onto a cookie sheet
- Lightly spray broccoli with cooking spray (so the salt sticks to it)
- Sprinkle salt to taste

Yes, this snack is pretty much all carbs, with a little fat and protein, but remember that dark green veggies like broccoli are negative fat foods so the more you eat, the leaner you get!

CLOSING REMARKS

Remember that even though this is the most current and most effective program to date, it is only as good as your own consistency. If you are following both the brain exercises and physical workouts with 212 degree intensity and commitment, it will deliver results beyond your wildest dreams. Believe in yourself and tell yourself you can do it! Program your mind for permanent success. Remember what the great Henry Ford said:

"Whether you think you can or you can't, either way, you're right."

Edwards Brothers,Inc!
Thorofare, NJ 08086
17 June, 2010
BA2010168